To Yvonne
with Love,

Clive

x

A Way of Medicine and Life

Clive Barker

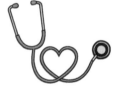

Illustrations by Emma Nissen

ISBN 978-1-909607-18-7

Contents

Dedication

For my family.

And also

friends, colleagues and patients,
who may be one and the same.

Foreword

As I lay in a bed on the cardiac unit of Chorley and South Ribble Hospital, feeling as if my heart was bouncing all over my chest, an intravenous drip of a powerful rhythm-stabilising drug feeding into my weedy arm, I thought: I don't really care what is done to me next, so long as I don't feel like this for much longer! At least I'd made it to the cardiac unit, which is more of a chance than some people get.

The next day, I was cardioverted (electrically shocked) back into a normal heart rhythm.

I wasn't supposed to be on the receiving end of treatment like this! I was a reasonably healthy 58-year-old who ran marathons, and tried to work hard looking after other people. What was going on?

This book is an attempt at an explanation.

Introduction

Twenty years ago I wrote and self-published a book for family, friends and colleagues, called *A Way of Life and Medicine*. By that time I had been a GP for over 10 years, and now it seems naïve and possibly conceited for me to have thought that I knew enough about what it took to live life as a doctor, husband, father and son to write a book. I am still learning.

I've had lots of highs and some lows. To others, they might not seem extraordinary, but to me they were special. This life and these experiences are the only chance I've got. YOLO – you only live once – as our lads would put it. I want to make the most of it, and leave a little record. *A Way of Life and Medicine* was my first such undertaking.

In the General Practitioner Writers Association's *How to… Guide*, the publisher wrote about that first book:

Clive Barker who is still a young GP has recorded graphically his training and his career experiences to date, such that Tina Ambury in a review commented: 'I feel it is a warts and all picture of the road to and through general practice. I gave my copy to my 15 year old niece who is keen to be a doctor. At least that way she will see how things really are for most GPs.'

Dr Ambury went on to be a vice chair of the Royal College of General Practitioners – though not directly as a result of reviewing my book, as far as I am aware. She also suggested my work was 'cathartic'. Looking back at the first book I think I learned more from writing it than I realised at the time.

Twelve years after the first edition of *A Way of Life and Med-*

icine was published I had run out of copies to give away, and quite a few people were asking about it, so I did have more printed, and by then, having a little more confidence than the first time, I also gave copies to patients who had enquired about it.

It has been fun, at least for me, looking back over the last 20 years, and during that time I knew I was going to write another book. I therefore have hundreds of scribbled notes stuffed into little diaries, which I have unfolded, deciphered and transcribed into this, my second and presumably last book, *A Way of Medicine and Life*.

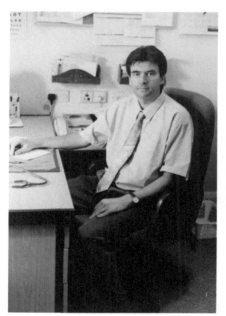
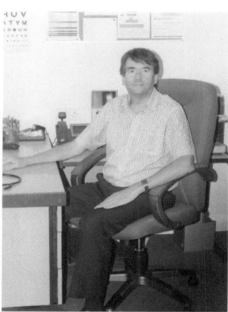

In my surgery 1996   *Still there 2016*

1. Physician, Heal Thyself.

'Has someone left a nappy in here?' tactfully asked Doreen, one of our hardworking receptionists, as she entered my surgery room to collect some papers early one morning.

'Yes, I've noticed a strange smell too,' I replied, not mentioning that this was uncontrollable flatulence emanating from me, having contracted giardia lamblia gastroenteritis on the holiday I had just returned from.

Danny, one of my great friends from university, and I had been on a skiing holiday in Andorra, each with our eldest two children, Joe and Matt (Danny and Jane's), and Tom and Adam (mine and Carole's).

We'd had a great time watching the lads who were seven and nine years old learn quickly, while Danny learnt more slowly, and I learnt at a snail's pace, unlike my skiing itself, which was out of control: fast. I was hampered by my fear of re-dislocating my left shoulder halfway up a mountain. My shoulder had regularly dislocated ever since my first year medical student friends had buried me in the sand at Blackpool. When skiing, I would always fall with my left arm close by my side to avoid dislocation, which on one occasion, in the days before skiing helmets, meant that the first thing to hit the ice was my head. Danny said he could actually see the stars and little birds circling my head cartoon-like as I lay on the ground, while a proficient French skier whizzed past commenting 'ça va?', but not stopping to hear the answer.

One thing the boys and dads did have in common that holiday was gastrointestinal collapse. I'm not sure what the food hygiene rating of the inn we stayed at in Andorra was, but it probably wasn't helped by their having a huge, long-haired, bear-like beast, which I think was actually a Briard dog, in the restaurant at the hotel. We all contracted giardia, and Danny did even better than me at skiing holiday-associ-

1

ated bowel problems by contracting campylobacter gastroenteritis as well. Vomiting, and being almost incontinent up a mountain can affect one's skiing style a bit, but somehow we all managed. I asked if anyone in our group had any Imodium or any other anti-diarrhoeal agents, but the only other skier who volunteered she was taking anything was a lady who started the day with a large brandy and 5mg of diazepam (Valium). Her skiing style was distinctly laid back, in fact flat on her back half the time.

This was the late 1990s. Our family life was full on. Max was slightly too young to go skiing yet, certainly in my company. Carole, having far more common sense than I ever had, kindly, and wisely, stayed at home with him.

Apart from gastroenteritis I've had a few episodes of illness myself, which provided me with a good insight into what it's like to be a patient. I've never actually had single days off work ill, but I have had some episodes of other interesting illnesses, needing more than days off, in fact about 16 weeks in a total of 35 years. In my first book I covered my pneumonia which I was off with for four weeks, and my depression, which took me off work for a total of about six weeks, and in this book you will learn more than you want to about my hernias, my shoulder, my diabetes, and my heart.

Although I am sure that my occasional encounters with ill health have never affected my judgement when looking after patients, when researching for this book I have read for the first time in full since it was published in 2013 *Good Medical Practice* published by the General Medical Council (GMC). I have reflected on how well I have followed its guidance.

2. Working with Doctors. Working for Patients.

'The Duties of a Doctor Registered with the General Medical Council' are listed on the inside front cover of the *Good Medical Practice* booklet by the GMC. The first paragraph states that 'patients must be able to trust the doctors with their lives and their health'. This is quite a responsibility, though there are obviously many other professions who also have this duty, both in healthcare and other walks of life.

Perhaps in healthcare more than other vocations, the emphasis may be more in partnership with the people we serve. We have to listen very carefully to concerns and respond to them, and respect patients' rights to reach decisions with us about their treatment and care. In medicine and other areas of healthcare, including nursing and physiotherapy, there may be a number of options to choose regarding how to manage a condition or health concern. Over the years I've tried to involve patients more and more in their management, with the degree varying with each patient. If I asked some of our older patients how they think we should proceed, it wouldn't be unusual for the response to be something like 'well, you're the bloody doctor, you tell me!' Younger patients may already have ideas about what they think is happening and how they think they want to manage their health. This aspect of general practice is covered in Domain Three (of four domains in GMC guidance), 'Communication, Partnership and Teamwork'.

The first of the three other domains is 'Knowledge, Skills and Attitudes', which includes learning, and as doctors, keeping ourselves up to date.

Over the years our continuing postgraduate medical education has changed, and usually improved. Twenty years ago pharmaceutical companies sponsored weekends away at posh hotels. Lectures would take place in the mornings attended by hungover delegates listening to 'experts' who, not very coincidentally, described research papers where the treatment of choice turned out to be manufactured by the company sponsoring the meeting.

I just about recall one such weekend based at the Wordsworth hotel in the Lake District, where after a Saturday morning lecture a round of golf was played in glorious sunshine. We re-hydrated afterwards on enormous complimentary gin and tonics and then had a huge meal. During the night, it wasn't until my bladder was about to burst that alarm bells started sounding in my comatose nervous system. It was the closest I had come to wetting the bed for 40 years – since I was in nappies.

As I sat near the back of the Sunday morning lecture with a pounding headache, proceedings were briefly interrupted when my two golfing partners, Pete and Danny, staggered in and found the only two vacant seats. These were large wicker chairs at either side of the lecturer's screen at the front of the room. Then they both fell very obviously asleep.

Nowadays most conferences are not sponsored, though some would argue that while the pharmaceutical industry plays a vital part in healthcare, the influence of 'big pharma' is still too great.

Years ago, so long as one had clocked up 30 hours or so of postgraduate learning, that was enough. Since 2002 we have had annual appraisals, where we supply genuine evidence of our lifelong learning. Since 2012, every five years our appraisals are collated into revalidation, to show that our learning is broad enough to ensure we really are up to date. These appraisals include: audits; learning from significant events; and patient and colleague feedback. Part of the appraisal and revalidation drive came about following the horrendous acts of GP Harold Shipman, who in 2000 was convicted of murdering at least 15 patients. Whether appraisal and revalidation would have raised concerns earlier is debatable, but most medical professionals feel that while they do involve a considerable amount of work, they are worthwhile. I found my appraisers helpful and supportive over the years.

Domain Two, 'Safety and Quality' of the GMC guidelines, not only deals with one's own health, but also concerns about colleagues. 'Whistle-blowing' is a frequently used term these days, and it has become easier to raise concerns about individuals or organisations whose care in some areas may be substandard, though whistle-blowers can sometimes be met with obstacles and lack of support, as documented by 'MD' in the satirical magazine *Private Eye*, which I have subscribed to for decades.

The sentence in the GMC guidance which I have tried to follow most closely is on the very first page, on the inside cover of the booklet *Good Medical Practice*. This is: 'Make the care of your patient your first concern'. This may sound obvious, but all sorts of factors influence care, including the resources available to help someone, be they time-related, financial, logistical, or even political.

For example, in 2012 the British Medical Association (BMA) supported a day's industrial action by doctors, reducing routine but not emergency care. This was the first such action for decades in an attempt to try to persuade the Department of Health and the Government to listen to doctors' genuine concerns, particularly regarding pensions, as all earlier measures had failed.

Personally, I felt this was not the main concern and not what we should have been taking action over, even though in most doctors' opinions and my own, politicians had behaved unreasonably. A day's action would have meant my postponing surgeries, childhood immunisations and visits to vulnerable people, which I was not prepared to do, and I worked normally from 6am as usual that day.

In 2016 there was a 24-hour strike by some junior doctors regarding a working contract that was being imposed on them, significantly reducing income for some, and affecting working life. Opinion of doctors within the BMA was divided, and, following further debate, significant industrial action did not go ahead.

It is understood that money is limited for the NHS, but in my decades as a doctor I've seen that reducing the income of the dedicated doctors making up the future of the NHS is not the way forward. I have been around long enough to see countless millions of pounds wasted, both on one re-organisation after another, including management restructuring that de-stabilises systems within the NHS, and the costs of management consultants.

In 2009 the Government employed McKinsey Management Consultants, who suggested the NHS cut 1:10 jobs, including those of doctors and nurses, in an attempt to save money. The Government did reject the report. Perhaps it would have been better to cut 1:1 jobs of management consultants.

The fourth and final domain described in the Duties of a Doctor Registered with the General Medical Council is 'Maintaining Trust'. This includes handling of complaints, and though I was lucky enough not to be subject to a formal complaints procedure in my career, I was Responsible Clinical Person for Complaints in my last years in general practice at Library House Surgery, Chorley.

Our Practice Management Team, John, Patti and Simon, were skilled at supporting colleagues and patients when complaints were made and my job was to give clinical input, and try to support the colleague who was being complained about, and the patient and their family with their concerns. We didn't get many complaints. I performed an audit in 2014 and we found less than 0.0001% of patient contacts with the practice resulted in a formal complaint. Half of these were in areas in which most primary care teams struggle, such as getting through on the phone at busy times, and patients being asked to register elsewhere if they had moved out of the area, so these were systems rather than individual people being complained about. Considering we had around 16,500 patients on our list for most of the time I was a partner, this was a considerable achievement and showed just how well we got on with our patients.

In a relatively close-knit community, patients often helped each other, though occasionally they would fall out with us, or one another, holding heated arguments in the waiting room. Perhaps half a dozen times in 31 years I had to ask patients to leave, and on even fewer occasions than that, escort them from the premises because of aggressive or abusive behaviour or taking drugs in the toilets.

Twice actual physical violence was witnessed by our team and innocent patients outside the surgery and in the waiting room. On one occasion we had to separate two men brawling on the pavement. In a separate incident a man was fatally stabbed in the road running by our surgery, the assailant then coming in to the waiting room and handing the knife to one of our senior receptionists.

In this latter event one of the people involved was our patient. This was obviously terrifying for those who witnessed what was happening, yet our brave team's main concerns were trying to resuscitate the dying man, protecting each other and our patients, and consoling those directly affected.

On the less traumatic occasions when we addressed complaints we also pointed out that people were at liberty to take their concerns to the NHS Ombudsman if they didn't feel their concerns had been resolved locally.

Some people resort to 'blame and claim' solicitors, even before accessing practice-based complaints procedures, lured by pictures of smiling, seemingly friendly faces and phrases like 'no win no fee'. Of course people should have a right to redress, and where appropriate, financial compensation, but medico-legal routes are very expensive, protracted, and usually adversarial, causing upset and worry to the patient or family concerned and to those healthcare professionals involved. Whether the UK will move to other systems such as 'no fault compensation' as in New Zealand, for example, is yet to be seen. In that system an aggrieved party is entitled to compensation without having to prove any other party was at fault.

My remit for this book isn't to go through each point the GMC makes, but it does make interesting reading, and details are available on line at www.gmc-uk.org. Although the last full update was in 2013, revised guidance is regularly published. It is essential reading for every doctor and medical student, and indeed much of it applies to other professionals in healthcare. I understand that years ago the GMC were seen to be less approachable by doctors and patients, though my limited experience when asking for guidance has been positive. I recognise that Fitness to Practice investigations are very stressful for all concerned. I did receive one letter from the GMC about 10 years ago in which they forwarded to me an anonymous handwritten letter which I think was from a relative (not a patient of ours) of a lady who sadly died, in which the author very explicitly wrote that I should have done more. The lovely lady herself, our patient for many years, even when poorly seemed as satisfied as she could be under the circumstances about her treatment. The GMC said that this was not a matter for them and it went no further.

While I was writing this book the GMC struck off a doctor who had, as encouraged in appraisal and revalidation, reflected in her appraisal about what could have been done differently in a tragic case where a six-year-old boy died from sepsis in 2011. These reflections indirectly affected her case, and this, and a growing number of other cases, according to an editorial in the *British Medical Journal* (*BMJ*) in February 2018, risks driving doctors towards defensive medicine, discouraging them from discussing errors, and denying health systems the chance to improve.

In the same edition of the *BMJ*: 'It is tragic that a child has died. But no one is served when one doctor is blamed for the failings of an over-stretched and under-staffed system. We must channel the sadness at [the child's] death, and the anger at [the doctor's] fate into positive change for safer patient care.'

A personal view in that edition, co-authored by two anaesthetists, was that: 'When we make mistakes, the pain of those mistakes can be unbearable. We search our souls, blame ourselves, and feel an enormous sense of guilt.' I can identify with that.

3. A Trying Husband and Dad.

Many patients became friends and during consultations people would kindly ask how I was, and my wife Carole, and our three sons Tom, Adam, and Max. I always had an up–to-date photograph of the four of them on one of the walls in the surgery which people would look at and comment how lucky I was. I was and indeed am lucky. It has even been suggested by serious colleagues in medical literature that such photographs are inappropriate in a doctor's surgery, because people consulting may not have been able to have a family or have lost loved ones. Our patients seemed genuinely interested in our growing family, and people often saw us out and about in Chorley town or Euxton village, where we live.

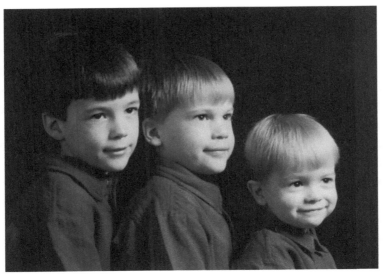

Tom Adam and Max, 1997/8

As the years went by, more and more people would enquire about my health, so much so I could have titled this book 'And how are you, Doc?'

The stoicism of many patients in the face of adversity is truly humbling. I would try to be empathic with people who might be going through awful times, when really I had little understanding, and no experience, of what they were going through, and here they were asking about me and my family's wellbeing!

Perhaps more people asked as time went by because I looked as if there was something wrong with me and, interestingly, a lot of people comment on how well I look now, possibly compared to the tired, pale, overweight version of me they saw at times over the years.

By the late 1990s Carole and I and the lads were well settled in our home which we had moved into in late 1996. We had lots of fun times with other young families, and would have been in a perpetual state of disorganisation and chaos as youngsters flew around our house and others', were it not for Carole's best efforts and those of Jane, our loyal part-time nanny who was with us for many years.

The lads were very successfully educated at one of the local state community primary schools, Balshaw Lane in Euxton, and then went onto Parklands High School barely a mile away. There they had a very good all-round education, both academically and in early life. Like most parents, Carole and I would rush to parents' evenings after work, standing in separate queues to try to get to see all their teachers. As an antidote to some of the seriousness of the work we had been doing, on one occasion I started suggestively eyeing Carole up and down in the parallel queue. I am not sure how to describe the expression she returned, but she raised her left hand and pointed to her wedding ring. As I was reasonably well known in the community by now, this caused some consternation in one or two nearby parents. Perhaps unwisely I joked to one of them that we have an open marriage, which took her rather by surprise. Fortunately we became good friends, though not in that way.

When our sons are home, some of the friends they made at school and college still visit us from time to time, which is special, having watched them grow up. One of them suggested that Carole and I must be 'swingers', as when he visited we would often be having dinner with one or two other couples. He's as wrong about this as his suggestion that I must have a massive 'schlong', because apparently our lads' friends can't see how someone like me could end up with someone as attractive as Carole.

As for the dinners, these are informal evening meals cooked with great finesse by Carole, and hindered by me. I am known for asking people round 'because it's our turn', and then contribute only by adding chaos while trying to help. Over 20 years ago we appeared on the television programme *Can't Cook Won't Cook*, and I was so bad we were asked back. Shortly after we appeared live in front of 3,000 people at the National Exhibition Centre in Birmingham on a version of *Ready Steady Cook*, where Carole was loudly applauded with her chef. Meanwhile my chef looked distinctly cheesed off to have been paired with me. My favourite recipe book these days is *Jamie's 5 Ingredients*, where, as the title suggests, only five ingredients are needed, and there are pictures of these ingredients individually, and then a finished dish as it is supposed to look, which doesn't bear much resemblance to mine.

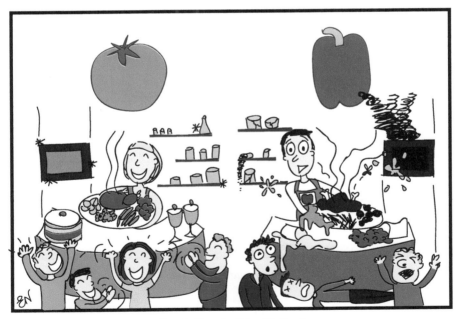

Ready Steady (Can't) Cook

Every now and then Carole and I would have a couple of days away, while willing grandparents or aunties would look after the lads.

Once a year I would go away golfing very badly with my friends Danny, Dermot and Richard, usually to Morfa Nefyn on the Lleyn peninsula in North Wales, where seagulls and the occasional seal would be lucky not to be hit by wayward golf balls.

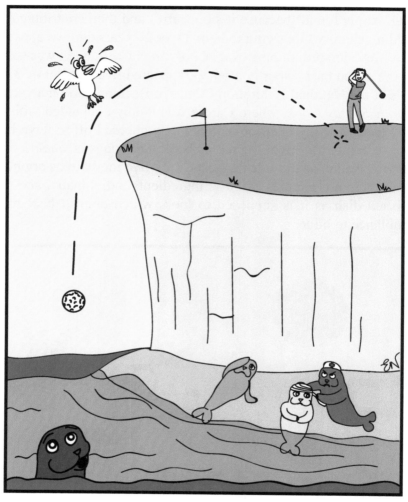

'Fore!' Endangered Seals

Occasionally Carole and I would go on separate holidays, like my skiing adventure. Carole would go with her mum and sister, or with a friend. On one occasion with her mother Barbara and sister Joanne, without me there to get them ridiculously early to the airport gate, their names were called out over the PA system, after which Carole insisted she must visit the Ladies, and was then escorted onto the plane by a man in a high-vis jacket. I would have been having kittens if I'd been with her.

We were lucky to have holidays as a family of five including in Croatia not long after their War of Independence, and in Florida six months after 9/11. People asked if we deliberately took our young children to zones which had recently seen conflict or disaster, which we did not, but we hope some of the places we have taken them to have made them realise how fortunate we all are.

As anyone who has been to Florida and the theme parks will know, this has to be organised with military precision. My obsessionality went even more over the top, constantly checking and re-checking we had all the documents and tickets. I re-checked our Universal Studios tickets so often that on one occasion they must have fallen out of my pocket, and when I arrived at the entrance on our first day, they were nowhere to be found! The lads looked up expectantly at me, and the nice lady at reception must have recognised I was about to burst into tears, believed my sorry tale, and, after taking a copy of my passport, gave us replacement tickets. We had a great time, and went on all the rides from Doctor Seuss to Jurassic Park, though at the age of barely five years Max was understandably anxious about Jurassic Park beforehand, but we still have a photograph of his beaming smile shining through his water-soaked face paint afterwards. For some years following, whenever we had the occasional disagreement he would accuse me: 'And anyway, you took me on scary rides'.

Closer to home we went to London, and to the Natural History Museum. One of my earliest memories as a child was going to London with my dad, on a plane, which actually had propellers. I was seven years old. I think we spent most of our money getting there, because we stayed at the YMCA (yes it was fun to stay there), and I don't know how we got back, but it wasn't on a plane. However, we did visit the Natural History Museum, which was awesome. Determined to try to instil the same sense of awe in our children we walked for some way to get to the museum for opening time. I couldn't wait to see the looks on the lads' faces as the doors opened and there would be Dippy Diplodocus, just like when I was there 40 years before.

Sure enough, there he was, dwarfing the five of us in the huge entrance hall.

'I want to go to Spar,' said Max. Spar shops in North West England were selling chocolate Kinder eggs with little toys in them and Max enjoyed these.

'But, Max, this is the Natural History Museum,' I tried to argue, to little avail. Since information and learning can now be brought electronically into our homes, it seems that museums sometimes don't hold the same fascination as when I was young. Having said that, nor do Kinder eggs to children in the USA, where my brothers still live. Apparently Kinder eggs have been banned from sale in case young children ingest or inhale small toy parts. Adults can still buy automatic weapons legally, which could kill dozens of children, but not a Kinder egg!

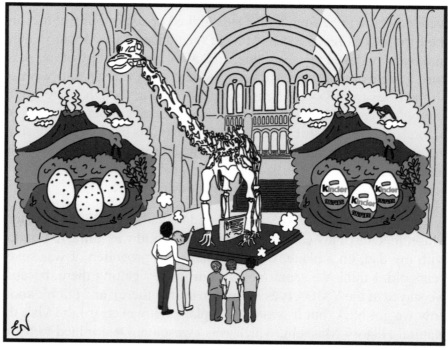

'I want to go to Spar'

When not on holiday we still had lots of trips out. I enjoyed, and still enjoy, live music. The Spice Girls were so good I even took

Tom and Adam. S Club 7 (I knew that Rachel Stevens had talent even before she appeared on *Strictly Come Dancing*), and Steps were fun too!

Musically, I've been stuck for most of the time in the 1970s, my adolescent years. Since most of the bands I was into then have split, retired, or died, over the last 20 years I have attended a number of tribute bands, some of which are very good. One of the most authentic visually is a band called The Musical Box, who recreate the shows Genesis performed in the early 1970s when Peter Gabriel was the lead singer. Some of my friends come with me and some others tease me mercilessly about my tastes, declining my invitation, saying they are washing their hair or cutting their toenails that night. Apparently Peter Gabriel took his own children to see The Musical Box some years ago, who then said to their father, 'If you could make a living doing that, then there's hope for all of us'. The set does consist of long songs up to 23 minutes in duration, after which the crowd cheers appreciatively, perhaps because they're relieved it's all over and can go for a wee, as most of the audience like me are ageing men with impending prostate problems.

Seeing what's left of The Who was great; Roger Daltrey at the end saying they hope to see us again, but couldn't be sure as they (ageing rock stars) were 'dropping like flies'.

Occasionally I'd go to gigs where the band and the audience aren't all ageing men, including Muse, Green Day (sorry about the air guitar, Max), Blink 182, and some years ago My Chemical Romance. I saw them with Max, my friend Paul, and his son Max's friend Oliver. Paul commented that he thought he was the only one in the Manchester Arena with grey hair, though at least he has hair. One brave young man was at the concert in a wheelchair, with total alopecia, possibly on chemotherapy, wearing an MCR tour t-shirt with F*** cancer on it (only without the ***s).

Over the years, Carole and I and the boys would go for walks in the local parks, especially Astley Park in Chorley and Worden Park in Leyland. The play areas were fun, and a lot safer than in our childhood. The lads and I would play football, coming home caked in mud.

Carole continued working really hard in the neo-natal unit and as a community neo-natal nursing sister. Jane was still a huge help, working very flexibly from early morning and sometimes until late evening. Carole and I would pass like ships in the night, yet as well as working Carole would run our home, bring up our lads, and support me in my by then 50–60 hours a week vocation.

I was pretty hopeless around the home. DIY was a disaster, and even now years later when trying to assemble something, while Max will stroke his chin and say 'Hmmm, interesting' I'll try to force it, saying 'Fit, you b*****d'. I try to have infinite patience with people but when an inanimate object won't go where I want it to or the computer crashes, I lose the plot. When a curtain rail wouldn't fit how it was supposed to I remedied the situation using superglue and dental floss. When I foolishly tried to plumb in a new dishwasher, the valve on the water input pipe somehow broke, so we had an impressive fountain spraying our kitchen. As I rushed into the garage to turn off the mains water, I found myself shouting, 'What a total f***-up', within easy earshot of our neighbours and patients.

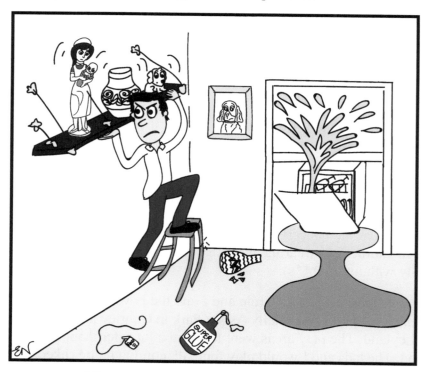

When multitasking becomes not tasking at all

16

As we approached the turn of the millennium I was very happy. Our kids were growing up healthy, our parents were still alive and well, and Carole and I had satisfying careers we enjoyed much of the time.

Carole achieved a 2:1 honours degree in Neo-Natal Nursing, and to my eternal shame, I was so wrapped up in work I didn't get time off to go to her graduation. Her parents, Bert and Barbara, did go, but I now find it incredible how I must have lost my sense of priorities. In fact, I have her graduation photo by my bedside table, so it's the first thing I see every morning.

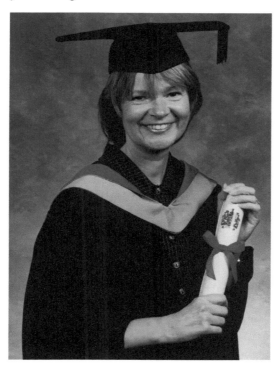

Carole's graduation, 2000

I have tried to show my appreciation for Carole over the years and in our early years I occasionally bought an appropriate piece of jewellery or something Carole was happy to wear. These have been outweighed by my blunders, which have made me rather less confident. Shortly after moving into our home in Euxton, Carole broke her ankle, which I misdiagnosed, and then I left the brake off the wheelchair outside A&E so she nearly ended up breaking more than her ankle. I bought her a lovely gift box and inside thoughtfully packed it with all sorts of useful items such as Vitamin D capsules, calcium tablets and an ankle support. Carole rummaged through these hoping to find the real present underneath, but unfortunately that was it.

I bought her a brooch with five semi-precious stones in it, to represent the members of our family, which would have looked reasonable on my grandmother, but not on someone youthful.

I found a lovely doll's house in a charity shop, fully furnished inside and with electricity to the lights.

The toilet seat even went down. I thought this would be a peaceful haven for Carole to retreat to when the maleness in our real lives got too much, but Carole saw this as another house to clean!

When walking in Worden Park more recently I saw an impressive set of wooden stocks for sale complete with hand holes and lock. I asked the woodworker if it could be engraved with the words 'For Carole's naughty boys'. After an initially quizzical look, he said he did know someone who could do this. Three months later he informed me that the engraver had been admitted to hospital under the Mental Health Act so couldn't help. I hope this wasn't as a result of my request.

With appalling and insensitive timing I brought the stocks home two days after we had been to see the film *Twelve Years a Slave*. They are now hidden in the garden.

Perhaps my worst attempt at trying to buy something useful was to get Carole a brand new set of gleaming ultra-sharp kitchen knives for Christmas, and then a hand-held Dyson for her birthday five days later. The lady in the Dyson shop said, 'This will be very useful for your wife, to vacuum up the parts of your dismembered body she's used the knives on.'

4. Pillar of the Community?

Some young doctors say they want to go into general practice for the work–life balance. I hope this works, but it is not always achievable as a GP Partner. In fact, some doctors think the GP Partner model will end soon, as many young doctors do not want to commit to a whole career usually in one place, possibly buying into the premises, and mopping up all the work when others have gone home. I can understand that view, but being a partner does give great stability, your practice being a place you can orbit around in all sorts of adventures, and still come back to.

Other options for a career in General Practice are available, including being a salaried doctor, usually in one practice, with all the clinical work but fewer of the business aspects. Many doctors work as locums, covering maternity or illness leave, often in different practices. Some doctors are GPs with special interests [GPwSI], combining regular GP work with dedicated clinical work such as dermatology or minor surgery. 'Portfolio' GPs are becoming more common, alternating GP work with, for example, hospice, sports, or occupational medicine.

I was lucky enough to be part of a great team of 50 people by the time I left. They would bring me back to earth when I lost focus. I recall saying to one receptionist, Lesley, 'You sound so cheerful when you're giving me extra patients to see.'

She replied, 'Well, there's no point both of us being miserable.' I hope I wasn't miserable often, as the positives massively outweighed the negatives.

After my crisis of confidence in the early 1990s (documented in my first book), I began to feel I could, after nearly 15 years, do this job of being a family doctor quite well. I'd got to know people, and they'd got to know me. When I knew I was going to write a second book, I wrote some quotes down from patients.

A man who had difficulty speaking after a stroke just managed to get out with great effort, 'How are the boys?'

A patient with dementia who couldn't remember much about recent hours or days said, 'I do hope your family are all right.'

It was wonderful to be part of a community. We were part of their lives, and they were part of ours. I got less uptight about our privacy, as most people were not intrusive.

It is less common now for GPs to live in the immediate vicinity of where they work, in their practice catchment area. In my early years I had been reticent about being seen in local pubs or restaurants, but then I recognised that people realised we were only human, and so long as we were focussed and completely capable of doing our job when at work, it was okay to be seen to be relaxing. Occasionally I would take this too far.

We used to frequent an excellent Chinese restaurant above a traditional English pub. Although it was permitted to buy pints of hand-pulled bitter from the pub and take them up to the restaurant, the lady who ran the restaurant seemed to disapprove of this, possibly because some guests like myself would consume too many pints of Theakston's or Timothy Taylor's Landlord. On one evening I stupidly asked if she would mind if we took the chopsticks home, to which she understandably replied, 'Sir,' (sarcastically), 'if this was an English restaurant would you ask if you could take the cutlery home?' In the same restaurant, where I thought I was a master in the use of chopsticks after my weeks in Japan many years before, a 'laundry charge' appeared on the bill, for £3. I thought this was rather unusual, but paid it anyway, and we departed leaving much of my four-course banquet on the table, my chair, and the carpet.

When our practice manager, Kathy, retired, we went on a Boatel cruise on the Leeds–Liverpool canal. I recall that it was a Friday and when driving around my home visits that day I passed a fancy dress shop. I called in, explaining that we were having a nautical party, and hired what purported to be an American naval officer's uniform, crisp bright and white, rather like the one Richard Gere wore in *An Officer and a Gentleman*. This was not a fancy dress party, but I wore it anyway.

Well into the evening, the Hot Chocolate song 'You Sexy Thing' was played, which had been made popular again by the film *The Full Monty*. With a little encouragement as we chugged along the Leeds–Liverpool canal with most of our work team there, I was loudly encouraged to re-enact the striptease scene from the film. Grabbing one of the menus, I opened it and said 'I have here a copy of the partnership agreement, which states that if any partner behaves in such a way as to bring the practice into disrepute, he will be expelled from the partnership'. (This was actually a clause in the partnership agreement when I joined).

'What do we think of that?' I said.

'Rubbish!' came the unanimous reply. I then proceeded to do a very bad impression of Robert Carlyle and his mates in the film, getting as far as my underpants, then legging it into the toilets to get dressed again. I understand there may be a video in circulation, but fortunately it didn't circulate in my years as a practising GP, and thank goodness this was in the days before social media.

5. Expect the Unexpected.

At work I made sure I was as alert and sharp as I could be. I will never forget a three-year-old girl coming into my surgery carrying a box of chocolates, accompanied by her mum. I had seen her three weeks before as an emergency, after she'd suddenly become acutely unwell. As I examined her a faint rash began appearing before our eyes, petechial, like tiny pinpricks. This was meningococcal septicaemia. I gave her intramuscular penicillin, after failing to access her small veins initially, and arranged an emergency ambulance to take her to hospital. After a stay there, she made a complete recovery.

We got to see the local geography of our wider community, working for our 'out of hours medical co-operative' to cover neighbouring practices and our own. I was fortunate that shortly before I started as a GP Partner, this organisation had been developed by local GPs, and we worked from a local base where patients could be seen or spoken to, and when visits were needed we had a fully fitted-out car and drivers who would navigate us there, often retired police officers or fire-fighters.

A dedicated team of receptionists and telephonists would organise the out-of-hours service. We were busy, covering a population of over 150,000 people, but with good planning to ensure sufficient medical and support staff were working at any one time, the emergency care was recognised as among the best in the country.

Night shifts were the most nerve-wracking. Often going out into the countryside to people we didn't know, who may be so unwell it was difficult to obtain a clear medical history, was a challenge. Dimly lit homes, sometimes with blue hazes of cigarette smoke, with slavering dogs present, made the diagnoses all the more difficult.

Nowadays, all young doctors work for at least four months in general practice, but decades ago some of them had little or no experience of medicine in the community. It was therefore frustrating, when trying to admit a patient, to be asked on the phone by a junior doctor who was in a brightly lit, warm, sterile (hopefully) hospital, 'Have you done a rectal examination?' (For example, if gastrointestinal or prostate diagnoses were being considered). Attempting this on a patient's sagging bed would probably have involved the GP falling into bed with the patient, and wouldn't alter the fact that the patient needed hospital assessment anyway.

Perhaps the most fortuitous night visit I was called to was a lady in her thirties with reported symptoms of abdominal pain and vomiting. We intended to visit as soon as practical, as we were on our way to visit a youngster with probable croup. The parents of the youngster then kindly phoned to say he had settled and was breathing comfortably, and they felt he didn't need seeing now, but would call back if they were worried.

We therefore went straight to see the lady who, when I arrived, was the same colour as her white bed linen, and barely conscious. I managed to get some history, including the fact that she had missed a period and that the pain was on one side of her lower abdomen. Her pulse was faint and rapid and her blood pressure unrecordably low.

She had a ruptured ectopic pregnancy. We called an emergency ambulance, and I gave intramuscular Adrenalin to try and increase her blood pressure, and on arriving at hospital her haemoglobin (red blood count) was 3.6 (or 36 in today's units), the normal being over 10 (or over 100 today).

She survived and made a full recovery, though understandably she was traumatised by the whole experience, as was I!

Home visits, though not often as dramatic, can keep you on your toes. I've only been assaulted once, by a cat! I called to see an elderly lady who was chesty and very breathless. She was sitting in a large armchair, and I let myself into her home, as instructed earlier by her carer, who had now left.

A medium-sized ginger cat sat placidly on the back of the armchair, looking at me suspiciously. After taking a medical history, halfway through the examination I asked the lady to lean forward and asked permission to lift up the back of her blouse so I could listen to her lungs. At this point the cat lashed out at my stethoscope-holding right arm, where it made three impressive claw marks. I leapt backwards and very nearly swore with surprise. The cat stared at me, daring me to try again.

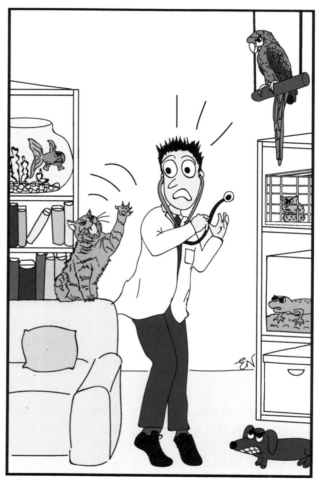

'Oh, don't mind the animals, they're harmless'

I'd forgotten one of the basic rules of home visits. Even if the owner of a pet says that Satan, the slavering teeth-baring Rottweiler, wouldn't hurt a fly, ask for the pet to be shut in another room. Even if a pet is usually harmless, it will not be used to a stranger walking in and examining its mistress or master who is in a vulnerable position and possibly in pain or other distress.

Still, pets make for wacky consultations. One of the most amusing must be with my friend Ewan, a GP in Anglesey, who when visiting a lady couldn't get her large parrot to shut up unless he talked directly to the parrot! Anyone passing and seeing the respected local GP taking a medical history from the parrot would have thought it wasn't just the lady who needed help.

Home visits, though time consuming, can give a healthcare professional a better idea of how someone is coping, and how their medical condition is affecting them (and their pets). Often a thorough medical history and detailed examination can be initially unremarkable, but on being asked to stand and walk a few steps, a patient can't. So getting to the toilet or making a drink is impossible, and this is where a multi-disciplinary healthcare team can be invaluable trying to help someone in their own home.

In trying, and usually failing, to be time efficient, before setting off I used to phone some of our elderly patients for whom a visit was being requested.

A frail person can seemingly take ages to get undressed and onto a couch or bed for an appropriate examination. I would therefore ask them by phone, in what might seem an unusual request, to take their clothes off from the area in question, and get into bed and I would be there in ten minutes. Hopefully this wasn't interpreted as 'Get your kit off, Doris and into bed, I'm coming round!'

On other occasions, with more haste than speed, I'd call at the wrong house, often unlocked, shouting in 'Hello, it's the doctor', much to the consternation of the resident who had not asked the doctor to call.

6. Boys with Toys and Pets.

Our home life continued as crazily as ever. The lads wanted pets, so we bought a hamster, which disappeared behind the fireplace (fortunately we didn't burn wood or coal), and went AWOL for days. After removing several bricks, we found her alive, but Hettie never recovered, so we bought a replacement, Harriet. She did okay until she developed a lower bowel prolapse. Seeing her in distress I picked her up to confirm what I thought was happening. She bit my middle finger with such ferocity, I have never screamed so loudly before or since.

The hamsters were nothing though, compared to the most evil animal I have ever had the misfortune to encounter: Blossom the rabbit. It was New Year 2000 into 2001 and Carole, Tom, Adam, Max and I flew to Fremantle, western Australia, to see Carole's brother Pete and his family; Annabel, Chantelle and Maxine.

It had been Carole's birthday the day before we flew, and I handed in a note I had written to the check-in lady. My note explained that Carole looks after the four men in her life wonderfully, and I would like her to have the opportunity to be upgraded to business or first class, as a birthday present, for a reasonable sum. 'Certainly, sir,' said the lady. 'That'll be two thousand pounds.' Carole joined us in economy class for the 24-hour journey.

We house-sat for a family my brother-in-law knew, who were away. All we had to do was look after the fish and the rabbit. The fish were a doddle, but Blossom was not. She used to stare out of her hutch looking at us just like Hannibal Lecter in *The Silence of the Lambs*. As instructed, every day we let her out to experience freedom, and every day, she dashed under the patio decking of the house and wouldn't come out. The lads bravely ventured under the decking and after an average of half an hour, during which they sustained significant head injuries, Blossom would be recaptured, only to fight another day.

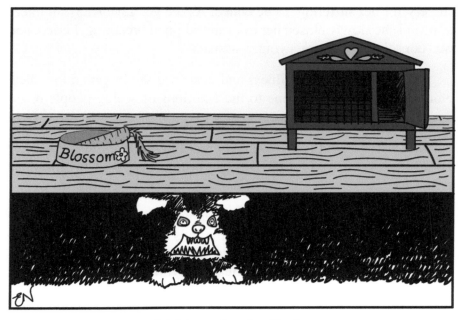

Bright eyes, burning like fire

Returning home from the blue, white and green of Australia, everything in North West England looked rather grey, but we got stuck in again, full on into our busy lives.

'We are not going to buy a dog today,' I said firmly, as apparently not put off by the Blossom experience, we set off to look at dogs.

Two hours later, we had bought a dog; Ruby, a King Charles spaniel. Ruby had had her third litter of pups some months before, and when Carole, Tom and I got her home, Adam was able to recognise her breeding days were over, exclaiming 'her tits are manky'. But she was great fun and game for anything. As one of my patients pointed out to me in surgery after seeing me jogging with her one day, 'Either you are going to have to slow down, or get a bigger dog!'

Ruby was a lovely dog who was part of our family for around six years. Sadly, she developed heart failure, hopefully not as a result of the occasional jog she did with me years before. At the end, she could barely walk, was breathless, and in obvious distress, and after discussion with Carole and the boys I took her to a local veterinary surgery for her suffering to be ended. As the vet gave Ruby an injection, and she slowly closed her eyes and stopped breathing, I cried, and was consoled by the vet's young assistant.

In spite of all the illness and death we see in general medical practice, we are not immune to the emotions of seeing people or indeed animals die.

Even without Ruby, we had great fun outdoors, while we lost all sorts of expensive toys the lads had been bought for Christmas and birthdays.

Replacing the screeching, bleeping and wailing noises of the toys that aunts and uncles bought the lads in their early years were remote-controlled models. These were exciting, until they went horribly wrong. My mum and dad bought a hybrid helicopter parachute, which on its third outing got caught by a gust of wind and ended up 50 feet high in a poplar tree in Worden Park, Leyland. I hailed a passing fire engine to see if they could help, but even their ladders didn't stretch that far. Three hovercrafts from Guy and Anne, at around £80 each, made their maiden voyage on Rivington reservoirs, only to be blown out of reach of the radio signal. It was March. I stripped down to my pants and swam out to get them to the sound of the lads singing 'there's only one Clive Barker' – which is just as well.

Carole and the boys and I joined our local gym, which also had an outdoor and indoor swimming pool. We all enjoyed playing tennis and badminton, though as the years went by the lads got better and better and Carole and I couldn't keep up, try as we might, which is of course the way things go.

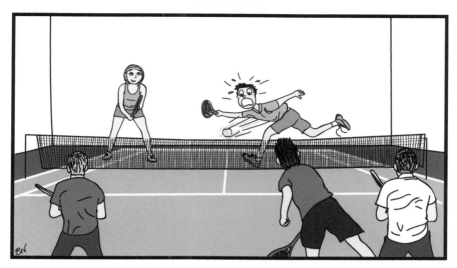

Game, Set and Match

One evening on the way back from the gym with Tom, the road under the railway bridge near our home was flooded. We stopped by the water, looked at each other, looked at the lake in front of us, and then I impetuously put my foot flat down on the accelerator, as if somehow by going faster we'd get through. The nose of my Rover II series dived into the muddy pool and we came to a dead stop right in the middle, water pouring under the door sills and engulfed in a cloud of steam like some kind of cartoon or slapstick comedy caper. A kind motorist towed us out and the next morning I phoned the AA, one of the three insurances I'm glad I've taken out, along with British Gas Homecare (as I am so useless) and mobile phone insurances when the lads lost them down toilets or in nightclubs, or in toilets in nightclubs.

The nice AA man in high-vis gear came out at 7am and amazingly got Rover going again. I'm sure I saw jets of water coming out of the pistons as the engine coughed back into life. The breakdown man kindly followed me to work or rather followed the cloud of vapour in which Rover and I were somewhere. When I told one of our senior receptionists about this she said, 'Boys will be boys'. When I told Carole what had been said, she, not unreasonably, pointed out, 'But you're supposed to be a man!'

There was an urban myth for months that a car had sunk in the floodwater under the Euxton Lane bridge. I think we may have inadvertently started this!

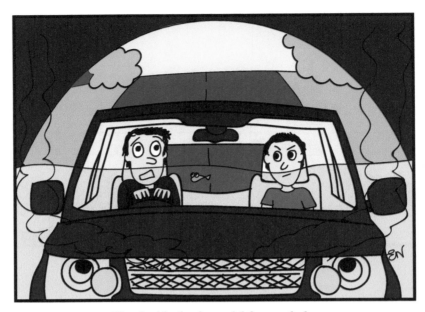

Not the ideal role model for our lads

The lads became increasingly interested in football, particularly Manchester United, and although I had seen this as a group of overpaid men kicking a ball around, it was quite therapeutic to watch Match of the Day on a Saturday evening or read the sports section of a Sunday paper the next day, before starting another busy week at work.

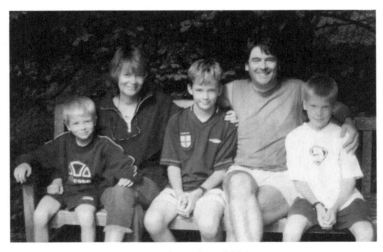

The five of us, 2001

7. Misunderstandings.

By halfway through my career as a GP I thought I was getting quite skilled at the consultation, which is at the centre of any doctor–patient interaction.

Many models of the consultation have been produced, but all depend on establishing a rapport between the patient and the doctor, and now, where possible, involving the patient in decisions about their care. I write 'where possible' because sometimes the patient may not at that time have capacity to be involved in certain decisions, through serious illness or severe learning difficulties, for example. I also use the term 'patient', but of course this is a real person, and not someone to be treated only as a patient with a set of symptoms or signs.

Listening carefully to the patient or their representative is vital. A patient of mine described a consultation with an eminent professor who held various offices, and must have had a lot on his mind, but our patient said that when this professor was with her, he seemed to give her 100% of his attention, even if it was for just five or ten minutes.

I have always tried, even with distractions like phones, computers or challenging previous consultations, to fix my attention on the patient I was with and to make it clear I was doing that. Explaining to the patient why you are asking certain questions, or why the doctor needs to examine the patient, helps to put that patient at ease and reduces the likelihood of misunderstanding or distrust.

This is not to say consultations always went smoothly. In the days when GPs still took cervical smears, I asked a lady how I could help after she had knocked and come into the surgery, and she replied in her Lancashire accent, 'It's smears.' I noted from her records that she had not had a cervical smear for some years, and to try to put her at her ease I explained that, while a pelvic examination was not an examination ladies particularly wanted, she had done the right thing in attending. This was also in the days when asking for chaperones was not always done, and it was thought that implied consent, by attending for a smear, was enough. I was almost at the point of asking if she would go into the examination room and remove her knickers, and cover herself with paper from the roll on the couch, when she started looking at me rather oddly. Picking up the non-verbal cue, I asked if there was a problem.

She replied, 'I said, "It's me ears"!' She was concerned about her hearing and I had almost asked her to undress and be prepared for a vaginal examination. Fortunately, after I apologised and explained my misunderstanding, she didn't report me to the GMC.

On another occasion I phoned up a lady to congratulate her on her new baby's safe arrival into the world. We GPs used to visit ladies post-natally and in fact got paid for doing so. Now we just don't have the time, but I still thought it good practice to phone to check all was well with Mum and Baby.

I asked her, 'How are you feeding Baby?'

There was a pause, then her reply: 'I'm feeling fine'. Then there was a pause by me, as I realised she must have thought I was the Austin Powers of the medical world, believing I had said, 'How are you feeling, baby'!

On other occasions I must have failed to introduce myself properly, including on the phone when one lady after several minutes asked when I was visiting to give communion, thinking she had been talking to her vicar.

Continuing in the consultation, once enough information has been gathered, and if appropriate an examination performed, a plan of action is formulated with the patient, in terms he or she can understand and make informed decisions about, be it a course of treatment, investigations, or often no specific action.

The patient must feel their concerns have been addressed and taken seriously. I say concerns, plural, because they may have several concerns about one issue or concerns about several issues. I think the record for me was a patient who attended a 10-minute appointment with a list of 13 different matters he wanted to discuss. Ten minutes – at present the usual length of a consultation, otherwise we couldn't see everyone who felt they needed to consult – is woefully inadequate. Suggesting a patient makes a further appointment to discuss other non-urgent matters can be a problem, as the patient may feel several are urgent, or that they have already waited a long time for their appointment.

Hidden agendas can be interesting on two levels. Patients sometimes consult with what appears to be a trivial symptom, and then, when hopefully the clinician has gained their trust, sometimes having taken over 10 minutes already, the real reason for the consultation, for example, erectile dysfunction, becomes apparent.

In recent years mobile phones and their camera and video facilities have helped consultations. For example someone may suffer from an intermittent rash, which may not be present when they consult, but if a photograph has been taken when it is florid, that is a help. I have also seen photos of interesting discharges from various orifices, organisms passed with a bowel motion, and bending penises. There is quite a common condition called Peyronie's disease, where due to a fibrous plaque in the penis, a bend is produced when erect. This is not apparent in the flaccid state people normally consult with. Hopefully patients don't accidently show these to acquaintances along with their holiday snaps!

The second level of hidden agenda I learned about when attending a GP tutor's course. In years gone by, medical graduate and to some extent post-graduate education, could be very hospital/specialist biased. A typical learning scenario would be that a patient would consult a GP, who wasn't able to diagnose their condition, so referred them to Outpatients. Effectively, what this seemed to say was, 'The patient saw their GP, but the GP was rather dim and had no idea what was going on. The GP referred to the clever hospital doctor, who did lots of fancy tests and treated the patient, who got better and lived happily ever after'. I think nowadays teaching is more primary care based.

Towards the end of the consultation it is important to ensure our patients have understood what has been explained or discussed and to 'safety-net'. Doctors have, by thorough history-taking and examination, put themselves in a position to make a diagnosis, but that diagnosis may not always be correct.

8. Uncertainty.

Where we earn our money, or our standing in the community, is not through the years we train or the hours we work, but in dealing with uncertainty. After a 13- or 14-hour day, going home thinking, 'I hope that unusual chest pain wasn't a cardiac problem', or 'I hope that child with what clinically was a viral illness wasn't the early warning of meningitis or septicaemia' is what weighs heavily.

If we admitted every patient to hospital when there was any doubt about the diagnosis, the NHS could not function and would be overwhelmed.

GPs usually manage risk very efficiently, but occasionally we are unable to foresee outcomes.

It would seem fitting to repeat the prologue from my first book here. It went:

The little boy looked up at me with trusting eyes. Earlier that day I had seen his father, who I thought had a brief self-limiting illness which would shortly resolve. Having explained this I said I would telephone in the evening to see how he was. I never got the chance. One hour after I had seen him he was dead.

Although that tragedy was to affect many people, it was to affect me in ways I could never imagine that day. In the months and years that followed I thought much about what one can and can't do in medicine, and in life, and in death. This book is a result. Everything in it is true.

That little boy with the trusting eyes grew up to be a fine young man, as did his brother. I am sure their dad would have been very proud of them, as was their mum.

It seems selfish to write about how I was affected, but without the love and support of my family, colleagues, friends, and patients, including that family who mercifully realised we don't always get it right, I don't know how I would have practised medicine again.

In subsequent years I would often phone patients, or families of elderly relatives or young children, between six and seven in the morning after I had seen a patient in evening surgery the day before. If their symptoms hadn't improved I would arrange to see them at the surgery or at home, or if they had worsened, admit them to hospital. The easy option would have been to admit them to hospital the evening before, but that was often not what the patient or their family wanted. It would add to the workload of the overstretched hospital team, and increase the risk of hospital-acquired infections and other complications.

Once in hospital people often have difficulty getting out. If there were adequate resources in the community, a medical assessment unit in hospital would be just that; a place where people could be thoroughly assessed, with appropriate investigations including urgent blood tests and ECGs and possibly X-rays or scans, and then discharged back into the community if safe, with support. Unfortunately support is often lacking. At a meeting I attended in 2015, it was estimated that in the Royal Preston Hospital there were 60 patients who medically did not need to be there, but because support after discharge was scarce, be it to their home or rehabilitation, or residential or nursing home care, they had nowhere to go, at huge emotional, and to the NHS financial, cost.

One way of reducing financial and emotional cost is to try to continue to care for people in their own environment, wherever that may be, if that can be compassionately achieved, and not admit them to hospital.

Several years ago I was asked to visit a residential home to see a poorly elderly lady with several long-standing disabling medical conditions. When I arrived, an emergency ambulance was in the driveway. Our patient had deteriorated further, so the carers had dialled 999.

'Mind you,' one of the carers said as I arrived, 'she wants to die.'

If that was the case, then unless she was acutely distressed, was the kindest action to call an emergency ambulance, with the prospect of being admitted to hospital?

I went to see another resident at the home. As I was leaving, the ambulance was still in the driveway. I asked if I could help. The paramedics explained that the lady was clinically dehydrated so they were setting up an intravenous infusion of fluids. I could see Chorley hospital, where she was eventually taken to, from where I was standing.

She died two weeks later, in unfamiliar surroundings, with unfamiliar carers, nurses, and doctors.

In recent years care plans have become more organised, with involvement of the patient where possible, and their family and carers. This needs to be discussed carefully and sensitively. 'Do not attempt cardio-pulmonary resuscitation' (DNACPR) forms can be completed if CPR is unlikely to be successful, or, if successful, the person's length and quality of life 'would not be of overall benefit to the person', for example in terminal illness or very old age or severe dementia.

One cannot of course generalise, and some people or their loved ones will feel differently from others.

Another situation where DNACPR forms can be completed is if there's an advance decision to refuse treatment (ADRT). Although I have never allowed my own personal feelings or opinions to influence patient care, these ADRTs can be helpful, drawn up when a person has capacity to plan for the future and followed when he or she does not.

I have an advance decision for myself at home, and in my medical records. As readers may know, I am very enthusiastic about life, but if and when the time comes that I develop severe chronic disease, I do not want intensive attempts to prolong my life.

DNACPR instructions and ADRT do not mean that a person is no longer cared for. Appropriate treatment and care to help the person and relieve symptoms or distress will be given, and patients and their families should be assured of this.

I saw a lady in surgery in tears, upset that she felt she had 'signed Mother's death warrant'. This is not what a DNACPR is. They are to try to ensure that frail and elderly people are not subjected to external cardiac compressions, which may break ribs and cause other trauma, including emotional trauma to the loved ones present, in a usually futile attempt to prolong life.

One does not go through a career in medicine, or hopefully any job, without being affected, and at times moved by seeing what people experience. As I said at my retirement evening, I'm not sure what the future of health and social care hold, but what I'm sure it shouldn't hold, unless a person has indicated otherwise, is very elderly, often demented people lying in nursing home beds, being 'fed' through a tube into their nose or through their abdominal wall, doubly incontinent, barely able to interact with their surroundings, existing, often for years. I've seen that many times, and it's heart-breaking.

General medical practice has changed in many ways in the years I was part of it. Some of it was easier in the twentieth century from a GP's point of view. Consultations seemed less complex, with fewer co-morbidities (one patient's medical conditions), fewer investigations, fewer treatments, and expectations not so high. Thus, there was less administration to be handled around each consultation.

Some of general practice was harder. My record for face-to-face consultations in one week was 249 patients.

One way general medical practice has changed for the better in recent decades is the expansion of the Primary Healthcare Team. In 1986 when I became a partner, there were doctors, receptionists, and secretaries. In the following years, in a leap of faith by our nursing colleagues, we appointed practice nurses, Jean being our first; healthcare assistants; and then nurse clinicians and advanced nurse practitioners; and, in the management team, a practice manager; HR lead; and IT/Operations manager. Each and every one plays a vital part in support of our thousands of patients, and each other.

9. Going for It.

In 2002, my mum, the boys' granny, developed a weakness in her left little finger. I thought this may be due to ulnar nerve entrapment at the elbow. Shortly after this she tripped over the bobbles on the approach to a pedestrian crossing. She went to see her GP, who referred her to a neurologist, who arranged neurophysiological tests. Dad and I were with her when the neurologist told her she had motor neurone disease (MND). One of Mum's first reactions to this news was her saying to the neurologist that if there was any treatment, and if it was expensive and not readily available, she would want someone younger to have the opportunity, rather than herself at the age of 67.

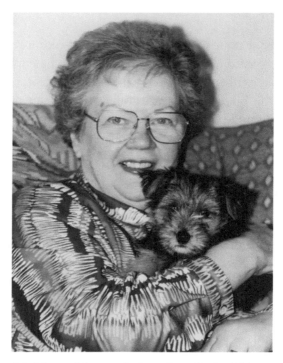

My Mum with carer's dog when she had Motor Neurone Disease, early 2003.

Over the next nearly two years, while she deteriorated, Mum was very brave and ably supported by Dad. They did obtain information about Dignitas, in Switzerland, but managed with excellent care from their GP, hospital and hospice team and the Motor Neurone Disease Association.

During 2003, what turned out to be Mum's last year, she encouraged us all to carry on living life to the full. In July, Carole, Tom, Adam, Max, and I met up with Pete, Annabelle, Chantelle and Maxine in Ko Samui, Thailand. We had a wonderful time – apart from Tom, Adam and I nearly dying.

We decided to go on a snorkelling trip to Ko Tao.

'As we set off, the weather was beautiful and the sea calm', as Tom and Adam wrote in their English GCSE exams years later, both getting 'A' grades for their essay question, which was something like 'Describe an horrific event in your lives where your stupid father nearly got you killed'.

I booked a boat trip with what looked like a reputable agent, and when we arrived we were escorted onto what appeared to be a large speedboat, with three powerful outboard motors on the back, so heavy that the boat was already out of the water at the bow. The three Thai crew made us welcome, and we got to know the 10 or so holidaymakers on the boat with us. We sped to Ko Tao, and had an enjoyable couple of hours snorkelling. Apart from a wave splashing my beautiful new digital camera, which fizzed, emitted a strange odour and then black smoke, and never worked again, our trip thus far was very enjoyable.

The crew were rather keen to get us back on board quickly for the supposed 40-minute journey back, because an enormous bank of black cloud was looming towards us obscuring the clear blue sky. Fifteen minutes after we set off the boat pitched and yawed in huge waves crashing all around, and the rain made it impossible to see where the sea met the clouds.

The safety equipment in the boat consisted of decaying 'life jackets', on most of which the fastening cords were snapped. Tom actually had an intact life jacket, and even managed to look quite cool sat diagonally opposite Adam and me, wearing a cap and sunglasses and with vomit dribbling down his chest.

Adam's life jacket was not complete, and as at that time he wasn't as experienced a swimmer as Tom, I tied him to me. He also was vomiting impressively, as were most of the passengers. Our confidence wasn't increased by the fact that the crew were looking increasingly concerned, huddled over their navigation equipment: a small hand-held compass. The father of a German family of four sat next to me with his head in his hands, repeatedly muttering 'this is crazy'. I had visions of a small section in a page of a national newspaper saying 'Father and two sons drown in Thailand sea'. Fortunately we did all make it back. When I said to Tom afterwards, 'When you take your kids, check the weather forecast first,' he replied, 'No, I just won't take them.'

Apart from nearly drowning I was fitter than I had been for some time by the end of our Thailand holiday. I was also pretty relaxed, partly due to the Thai massages available in the hotel gardens. Although almost painful at the time, (I drew a poor illustration of a dislocating shoulder to try to communicate 'please go easy on my left shoulder girdle'), I don't think I have ever been more relaxed. My metabolic rate was so slow that I meandered gently to the swimming pool where I lay face down in the water, and held my breath for my record of 4 minutes and 11 seconds.

Within days of returning from that holiday my brother Guy and I took part in the Salford Quays Olympic Distance Triathlon, a 1500 metre swim, 40 kilometre bike ride and 10 kilometre run, to raise funds for the Motor Neurone Disease Association. I borrowed a bike from a friend and Mum bought us a bike for Guy to ride, because she wanted to contribute something while she was still alive, as well as after she was gone. Through that and other events, thanks to the kindness and generosity of family, friends, colleagues and patients, over £15,000 was raised to support the good work of the Motor Neurone Disease Association (MNDA), and we're not done yet.

I remember seeing Mum in her lounge, sitting in her electric wheelchair with the head support, relaxing panpipe music playing in the background, knowing her life was nearly over. As her speech became less clear, she could still communicate slowly. Nevertheless, the frustrations of MND were evident, such as not being able to swat away a fly landing on her head.

The following poem was one which Mum poignantly related to during her last months.

To Blaise

(1975-1988)

Old cat on the sill

Sitting to gaze

Letting the sunlight fill

Your drowsy days

Watching the world slow down,

Content to dream –

Tell me, old veteran,

Does it not seem

That birds are swifter now

The trees more high

The mice more cunning than

In days gone by?

The garden – close

That was once so small

Is world enough, wide enough

To hold your all

Old cat on the sill,

Sleep in the sun,

Dream, for the golden day

Is almost done.

Mum died 27 December 2003, spending her last four days in St Anne's Hospice. She'd always been wonderfully stoical and up-beat, and enjoyed seeing our lads driving her electric wheelchair and saying, 'Ah, Mr Bond, I have been expecting you'. Monty Python's 'Always Look on the Bright Side of Life' played as we left the crematorium after a simple humanist ceremony.

Mum had said in her final months that if ever we were in doubt about doing something, 'go for it,' which we did, and still do.

10. Intelligent Life?

On the world stage, in 2003, many people were suffering not because of individual illnesses, but through the effects of war. I recall seeing the bombing in Iraq on television early one morning. The Prime Minister Tony Blair had experienced some political success in Northern Ireland, and former Yugoslavia, but I couldn't help thinking that while Saddam Hussein was undoubtedly evil, for Britain to take part in a coalition led by US President George Bush was madness.

Most of my generation in this country have been lucky never to have been the victims of war, but throughout my life it has seemed that there is always one people at war with another somewhere in the world, which is why I've been a member and supporter of Médicins Sans Frontières.

Occasionally over the years I have wondered whether I would be any help volunteering abroad, but my tropical medicine and surgical knowledge is such that I would probably be useless, or even worse, a liability. I hope I'm not just trying to assuage my guilt because I'm used to a cosy bed and toilet facilities and am unlikely to be blown up. The workers in these fields are true heroes, and all I do is subscribe to the charity, as well as to interesting journals including the *New Internationalist*, and the *New Humanist*, which again help me realise how lucky I am.

Sometimes I take myself too seriously and think about life, the universe and everything. I found a note I wrote to myself around 15 years ago, possibly after a glass or more of wine, trying to be profound.

The human race is possibly living in the most fortunate and opportune time there has ever been and ever will be.

Although there will be many things to discover yet, and although we are not able to help people in some ways as much as we will be able to in the future, for example with diseases yet to be cured, we have so much to be grateful for.

In another one hundred years the world may be over-populated and over-heated and unless we come up with new ways to produce energy, we have more resources now than we may have in the future. Why are we still fighting wars, and being so destructive, yet when peoples work together we can achieve so much?

As Monty Python sang:

So remember, when you are feeling very small and insecure,

Just remember how amazingly unlikely is your birth,

and hope that there's intelligent life somewhere out in space,

'cause there's bugger all down here on earth.

My family and I have been very lucky to see something of the world, party spurred on by people like Michael Palin (of Monty Python), who, when asked what was the most important thing he'd learned from his travels, said something along the lines of: 'When one travels around the world, one realises the peoples of the world have much more that unites them than divides them'.

Another of my heroes who has travelled the world and taught us so much about it is Sir David Attenborough, and although I am not an avid reader or television watcher, I would keenly read or watch any of the amazing BBC series about our earth and life on it. My favourite shop is Waterstones, and on one occasion I attended a book signing by the great man, so I could give my dad a copy, who in his way has been inspiring to our family.

Of course I can't claim that our trips were anything like as educational as the travels my heroes took. Particularly when ours were mainly unashamedly aimed at having a good time.

In 2004 we went back to Florida, the day after Hurricane Charley, when only one half of central Florida's three airports was left open. There was absolute chaos on our arrival, and knowing that car hire opportunities would be stretched, even though we'd booked one, I impetuously said to Carole and the boys that I would go to the Alamo car hire desk, if they could pick up the luggage when it finally came through tight security and meet me at the car hire desk. Three hours later, still standing in the Alamo care hire queue, the man queuing in front of me, Gary, and I had given up hope of ever seeing our families again, and almost started a bromance.

Carole and the lads, to whom I had forgotten to give any money for food or drinks as I charged off, had been searching for me in the Alamo car hire queue in the other terminal! Stupidly, I had not thought that there may be two such car hire outlets. Eventually, we met up, and drove through the night, crammed into the third last available car, a small Chevrolet, which seemed like the equivalent of an old Mini. Carole and I debated heatedly where on earth we were going, but fortunately our lads were mature enough to help, and we eventually found our holiday home.

Most of our holidays are like those in the *National Lampoon* series. I am aware, like Chevy Chase's character in those films, that I am an acute embarrassment to my family on holiday.

On that 2004 holiday I tried Disney's Summit Plummet 60mph vertical water slide, and my swimming trunks shot so far up my natal cleft my voice went at least two octaves higher.

On holidays in countries where English is not the first language, out of courtesy I try to learn some words and phrases, only to be met with uncomprehending quizzical looks, and then replies which I don't understand. Hopefully they are not along the lines of the pompous Parisian waiter in *National Lampoon's European Vacation*, subtitled, 'You are an ass, but your wife has nice tits'. Usually I resort to speaking in English slowly and loudly.

46

On one occasion in Spain I explained that I was in the medical profession myself to the Spanish doctor I was consulting with, and that all I needed was ear drops for my 'swimming pool' (infected) ear. She initially didn't believe I could possibly be a doctor, as I had squeezed half a tube of Savlon into my ear, trying not to trouble anyone.

All five of us went skiing once Max was old enough, or rather once I had decided he was old enough. He would have been fine years before, but after Tom falling and smashing his front teeth on our first holiday abroad as a family in Lanzarote, aged 18 months, when I was supposed to be looking after him, I was over-cautious. Until we got on the slopes, that is.

In Bulgaria, the nice man in the ski hire shop asked if we would like wax on our skis.

'Would that make us ski better?' I asked.

'Oh yes,' he replied confidently and, for what I assume was a very reasonable price, waxed Carole's skis particularly keenly, obviously impressed by her style in bright new and as yet untried skiwear.

This made her skis and the snow they were gliding over have a friction coefficient less than atomic particles, and made skiing almost impossible, though slightly easier after mulled wine.

I experienced a similar lack of traction in Austria, when sledging. My considerable momentum ensured I failed to negotiate a rather tight turn and literally took off over the edge of an Alp, ending upside down in a pine tree, with the salopettes I was wearing torn to ribbons. Tom had videoed my first attempt at Alpine gymnastics from the sledge behind, made all the more amusing in hindsight by him p***ing himself laughing.

Unfortunately, somehow, I lost the digital footage, which is a shame as I'm sure it would have won money on *You've been framed*.

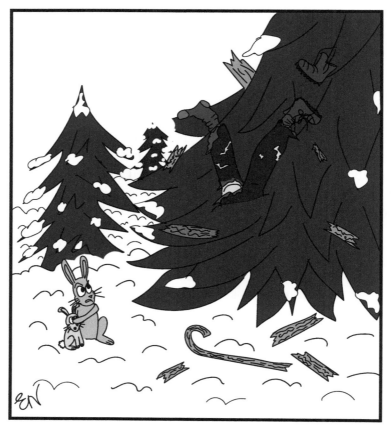

Alpine adventures

As well as taking part in most of these crazy adventures, Carole would patiently patch us all up ready for the next one. Thank goodness that as well as being an amazing wife and mum, she is also an experienced nurse.

She even managed to bring home pretty souvenirs of our trips, probably the most precious being a Lladró midwife, cradling a baby in her arms. She looked beautiful on our mantelpiece, until for some inexplicable reason a ball knocked her off, breaking her into a million tiny pieces. Carole was out at the time, so I rushed into Chorley to a jeweller's, where the lady behind the counter was one of our patients. I recall saying something like, 'I know I've never actually saved your life, but you can save mine!'

48

We ordered a replacement, but it was going to take days, and Carole is more observant than that. When she came home, even though we boys had tried to rearrange the ornaments on the mantelpiece to hide the gaping gap where the midwife once stood, she noticed. When she asked what had happened, probably the first sentence shouldn't have contained the word 'ball', after all the times she had not unreasonably asked us to refrain from playing with balls in her beautiful lounge. She went out for a long while that evening.

Needless to say the only souvenirs I've brought home from abroad are probably deranged liver function tests, and the occasional weird haircut. In America, visiting my brothers, Alec and Guy, revenge was wrought for the time I cut Alec's hair when I was four and he was two. As my best man Ewan commented at mine and Carole's wedding, and as was confirmed with a photo, Alec seemed to wear a balaclava for some time after that. I came back with a haircut performed by my brothers after only a moderate amount of alcohol, with a safety electric razor I must add, about which my senior partner at the time, Bill, asked, 'Did you do that for a bet?'!

Even on holiday, though, I never strayed too far from the serious side of important academic research. When on the Costa del Sol I gathered data for a project I completed on returning to North West England. The title of the subject was: Does San Miguel lager taste better when sampled with one's family in a Spanish restaurant overlooking the sun-soaked Mediterranean Sea, or outside the Laughing Donkey family pub on a grey Blackpool day waiting for your children to exhaust themselves on a climbing frame?

I think you can guess the answer.

11. Lifelong Learning.

After our holidays Carole and I returned to work, which for both of us was going reasonably well. Our Partnership had a couple of partners come and go, but the basic core stayed strong.

Medical partnerships can be harmonious, like ours most of the time, and indeed the majority of local practices worked well. Our wise senior partner said many years ago, not about any in our practice, that some people know the cost of everything, and the value of nothing. I'd like to think I've taken on board and benefitted from colleagues' insights over the years.

Patients seemed mainly satisfied with the service we were providing. On the day of an audit by the Primary Care Trust, one of our patients said, with perfect timing, 'You make us feel we're not just numbers.'

We enjoyed teaching medical students, and I was at that time approved as a GP Trainer. In this role doctors who had spent three or more years in a variety of posts since graduating, and now wanted to be GPs, would spend a year with us, just like I had 20 years before. At that time we couldn't lose any clinical time consulting with patients, so this was in addition to all my usual work. After a successful year I didn't continue as a GP Trainer, because to do it properly while not dropping any of my usual clinical work was not practical.

Now one of the other partners is a GP Trainer, and Library House Surgery has Foundation Year 2 doctors attached with us for four months each, in their second postgraduate year. To have young doctors in training around is fun, and I probably learnt more from them than they did from me.

I occasionally visited our local children's hospice, Derian House, where youngsters with life-limiting illness and their families are supported. Seeing the kids there, including some of our practice's young patients with degenerative neuromuscular disorders, tumours of the central nervous system, bone cancers or metabolic disorders, made me realise how lucky we are, but also made me question how could these things happen, even with my scientific background. I sincerely hope that children and families find comfort in some sort of support or faith. Any religious belief I had was at most tenuous, and over my years as a doctor I believed less and less in any kind of religion.

I now consider myself to be a humanist. I fully respect any-one's belief, so long as they do not force it on anyone else, or use it as an excuse for extremism.

The God Delusion, by Richard Dawkins, and some other athe-ist literature, at times seems to imply that religious people are stupid or dangerous or both, which is of course absolutely not the case. My understanding that this universe started 13.7 billion years ago as an in-finitely hot, dense, pea-sized singularity is probably harder to believe than creation by a grand designer.

I have been honoured to be named as godfather to three special young people, and although I am hopeless at remembering birthdays and other significant events, it means a lot to be a part of their early lives.

While many families stayed close and supportive over the gen-erations, many consultations as a GP occurred because families were splitting up. There are all sorts of reasons why this happens, but it was sometimes puzzling why men, and less often women, leave their families. Over the years many seemingly good husbands, wives, and most importantly, parents, decide they need more 'me time', or find someone with whom they think they can be happier. The remaining parent would consult, having difficulty understanding what had hap-pened and in coping with being a one-parent family. The absentee par-ent sometimes leaves the remaining family in financial difficulties, not contributing to help those left behind. There were occasions when the person who had left their family would consult, racked with guilt, or wishing they'd never left; realising they had similar issues with their new partner; similar problems, worries, and the flaws that we all have. Often there was little medically I could do, and to see the effects on children of family break-ups was upsetting.

12. The Changing World of Medicine.

The early 2000s saw further change in the way primary healthcare was organised. Fundholding, which ran from 1990 to 1997, was abolished by the Labour government and in 1999 primary care groups were established. The idea was that, instead of individual practices buying services in fundholding, primary and community health services were brought together in a single organisation with a unified budget for delivering healthcare to local communities. Primary Care Trusts (PCTs) replaced the groups between 2001 and 2004. PCTs were managed by various directors who became members of a board, who were advised by clinicians, including GPs.

We have tried to adapt to the never-ending reorganisations over the years, and I have lost count of how many Secretaries of State for Health there have been in my medical career, and how many changes of Government there have been. All the while we have tried to provide continuity of care.

GPs' morale at that time was low, and there were difficulties recruiting and retaining GPs.

Our lives were changed by a new contract in 2004. The British Medical Association and other medical organisations negotiated a formula with the Government which rewarded primary care for achieving certain targets and providing services, including the Quality Outcomes Framework (QOF). Certain parameters were measured, for example, in the care of people with long-term conditions such as diabetes, ischaemic heart disease and chronic obstructive pulmonary disease.

The income of many GPs increased considerably, partly because targets were already being achieved, which the Department of Health and to some extent the medical profession hadn't realised. The press had a field day, reporting that some GPs earned over £100,000 a year, which at our surgery was not the case, not because we weren't providing good quality care, but partly because we continued to focus on patients' concerns and needs, rather than the number of points we could collect. Many patients nationwide would consult their primary healthcare professional, and instead of focussing on what the patient wanted to discuss, the consultation focussed on whether they'd had their cholesterol checked recently, how much they drank or smoked, and how much exercise they did, which, albeit important, detracted from the patient's focus in their 10-minute consultation.

Headlines such as *The Sunday Times* on 29 July 2007 which read: 'Official: Doctors do less work for lots more pay', biased public opinion against GPs, understandably – but inaccurately.

I wrote to the paper in these words. 'It seems ironic to be reading your report at 7 o'clock last Sunday morning, in between seeing patients. Whilst I and most of my colleagues feel privileged to help our communities in a relatively well paid position, we do feel recent articles in your and other newspapers are balanced against us.

'I work more than sixty hours a week in a responsible job where people's lives are at stake. We and our teams provide extremely good value for money, better than nearly all other primary healthcare services in the developed world, providing the vast majority of healthcare for a small proportion of the total NHS budget. It costs the NHS 20p per patient per day to receive care from their GP practice, less than it is possible to insure a pet hamster for veterinary fees!

'Whilst in the last two years my income has increased, it is not to the huge sums sometimes quoted in newspapers. The reason for the increase is that government did not realise how hard we had been working for the last twenty or more years, and that we were already doing most of the work we are now being paid for.'

The UK spends a smaller proportion of gross domestic product on healthcare than other comparable European nations, and primary care at that time received less than 10% of that funding, with little increase since.

The GP Contract allowed individual doctors to opt out of out-of-hours care (from 6.30pm to 8am), and PCTs commissioned out of hours and other services. I continued working for Chorley Medics, as I felt it was important to keep up to date with emergency care in the community. Every few Thursdays I would work from 6am to 7pm, come home and go straight to bed until 11pm and then get up to work from midnight to 8am. I wouldn't officially work after that on a Friday, but sometimes there were administrative duties such as contacting a patient's usual GP, or trying to help with death certificates (so someone didn't have to have a post mortem), which could take up much of the Friday. In the evening I was knackered, falling asleep in front of the TV with a San Miguel lager by my side.

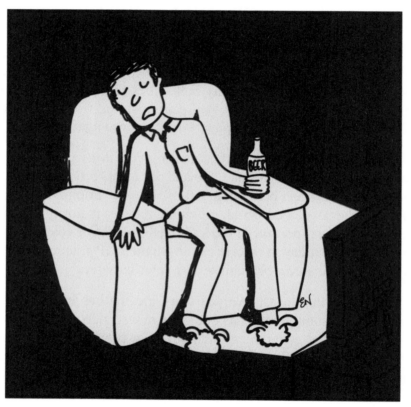

Relaxing on a Friday evening with a mate, San Miguel

As most practices became 'paper light or almost 'paperless', at least entries were legible, and in most cases more organised.

As QOF templates developed, while sometimes distracting from the consultation, it became easier to document certain criteria and to extract data for statistics and audit. One audit I did was to see how my computerised records compared to my written records, and because of my relatively slow keyboard skills my computerised consultations consisted of only two thirds of the words of a written consultation.

As an antidote to my rather dry recent section on NHS organisation, the following are excerpts from written notes up to the early 2000s; not from our practice, I am relieved to say, and although I have not seen them first hand, I have read them in both the *GP Writer* journal and the journal of the Medical Protection Society.

Most of these are mistakes in spelling or grammar or have been dictated but clearly not read, and the last one is an example which, no matter what your opinion of a patient or family, you do not write in medical records.

- The baby was delivered, the cord clamped and cut, and handed to the paediatrician, who breathed and cried immediately.

- When she fainted her eyes rolled around the room.

- The patient has been depressed ever since she began seeing me in 1983.

- The patient is a 79 year old widow who no longer lives with her husband.

- Between you and me, we ought to be able to get this lady pregnant.

- Rectal examination revealed a normal sized thyroid.

- Both breasts are equal and reactive to light and accommodation (to non-healthcare readers this should refer to the pupils of the eyes).

- The patient lives at home with his mother, father and pet turtle, who is presently enrolled in day care three times a week.

☐ The patient has chest pain if she lies on her left side for over a year.

☐ I've met the patient, the wife, his children and the pet rabbit. Of the lot of them, the rabbit is the most intelligent.

When dictating routine letters which are not particularly fascinating, I tried to make it more interesting for me and our hard-working secretaries, for example by dictating whole sets of letters in a Scottish accent, or extrapolating the normal 'I would be grateful if you could see this (patient)'. I worked up to 'I would be delighted if...' (consultants were more delighted with their letters if it was a private referral), to 'I would be sycophantically ecstatic if' through 'It would give me multiple orgasms if...', finishing with 'It would be the greatest moment in the history of the universe if you would kindly see this patient'.

Only once in a referral did one of our secretaries not spot my tongue-in-cheek expression of 'I am not sure what's going on here, so I think I'd better refer to a cleverer doctor than me', and the letter was actually sent. Serves me right.

Our patients too had a great sense of humour, even in the face of adversity. One of our patients had a quite rapidly advancing cancer, and I phoned him to ask if it would be okay if I came to see him. Another of our patients, who was also a colleague and a friend, was visiting him at the time, and told me after he had put the phone down he turned to her and said, 'If he's coming to see me I must be bloody ill!'

Another of our elderly patients collapsed and died in one of the local betting shops. His wife saw me shortly afterwards, and although sad at his passing, said that it was how he had wanted to go. While never laughing at our patients, we would sometimes have a laugh with them. I emailed my partners letting them know our betting patient had died, and asked, 'What are the odds of that happening?' One of the replies was, 'Odds aren't being offered, because he was a dead cert.'

I am acutely aware that my IT and digital communication skills lag behind most of my contemporaries', although as soon as mobile phones became available I bought Carole one, larger than a house brick, because I was concerned about her being out alone nursing in the community. I've tended not to buy electronic equipment unless I've needed it. I have a simple mobile phone which is not a smart phone.

When Max's Apple laptop malfunctioned, and he went on his gap year, I took it to the nearest Apple approved store, and thought I was going to be ejected as an imposter. I walked into the bright white showroom and hesitantly presented myself at the reception desk where a tall young man looked down on me and may as well have said, 'Greetings, inferior humanoid, what are you doing here?' His hands then hovered over the keyboard while unintelligible images appeared on the screen and he arranged for it to be fixed.

13. Teenage Years and Four Boys.

By the mid 2000s our lads were growing up. Seeing Tom at his prom leaving Parklands High School with a pretty young lady on his arm made me realise that they were becoming young men. Carole was very patient with the three of them in her house: slightly spotty, moderately sweaty, and very itchy, if the amount of scrotal manipulation through pyjamas and trousers was anything to go by.

Carole refers to me as her fourth son, partly I guess because I try to follow J. M. Barrie's and Peter Pan's advice to 'become an adult, but never grow up', and not, hopefully, because I was too spotty, sweaty or itchy.

Around this time though, for some reason I developed swellings in my groins which were not supposed to be there. I subsequently spent my first ever night in hospital having my hernias repaired, and thanks to the skill of the eminent surgeon who performed the operation I have had no problems since.

We were lucky enough to have holidays in Greece and Turkey where the lads would go off with other young people in various activities and clubs, while Carole and I spent much valued time together.

These holidays, though worth every penny, cost a lot, so in 2006 we were persuaded to buy into a sort of timeshare. Over the years we have been lucky enough to have had some good holidays, but one of the things I have learnt is not to buy into a timeshare. Promised availability not materialising and escalating 'management fees' mean that this is not, as yet, value for money.

However, it would seem churlish to complain about holiday accommodation when thousands of people in this country and millions of people worldwide don't have a home to live in.

We have made some good financial decisions over the years, and others less wise. Buying the only two houses we have ever lived in were good decisions, even though they stretched us somewhat at the time.

Buying 'added years' to my pension was a good idea, particularly as no one saw the current pensions crisis coming at the time, 35 years ago. In fact, I feel very guilty that, for reasons I can't recall but suspect it was because we were all very busy working hard, I didn't get to tell my medical best friends about this, as they frequently now remind me. I vaguely recall my friend and house officer colleague Brian saying that I should buy some of these added years that effectively meant we could retire earlier on a better pension, which is part of the reason I can sit here in Adam's room on a Friday writing this.

Building Library House Surgery was a wise decision. In the early 1990s we rented part of a health centre, which became increasingly crowded and unsatisfactory to work from. Building premises for our own partnership meant we had more control of our working environment and significantly more space, though over the years we added two extensions as the primary healthcare team expanded. This move was particularly insightful of my then more senior partners who actually benefitted less than I did, both in time in the surgery, and financially on leaving.

One of the initially less wise decisions was having a posh bathroom fitted at home after a smartly suited rep visited, foolishly invited by us. He persuaded me that many thousands of pounds for this state of the art masterpiece was good value, when finances were tight.

To be fair though, the people they sub-contracted to do the work did find out that our house was a death trap.

Built in the 1860s, initially as a barn, research has suggested that it became possibly a ropery, then a car repair facility, and we do know that from the 1940s to the late 1970s it was a weaving shed, with six looms in it. The story goes that when the mill owner was told by Debenhams, for whom they used to make curtains, that in future they would be paid by the metre rather than the yard, but at the same rate, the mill closed down because that difference represented the profit margin.

Then some builders bought it and converted it into a family dwelling, though they seemed to run out of money, so then a couple bought it and spent at least five years further renovating and furnishing it. This obviously took its toll because then they acrimoniously divorced, and we bought it.

Many a workman has visited when something has gone wrong and said, 'Well, I've never seen it done like that before.' Our bathroom fitters found out that our house wasn't properly earthed, and when we phoned Carole's brother Mark, who is an electrician, he doubted that anyone would have been stupid enough not to ensure the house was earthed. Then, bless him, he was at our house within the hour, confirming that we weren't in fact earthed, and he hammered a huge copper pole into the ground and connected it to the house there and then.

We also found we had a gas leak which had been going on for an unknown length of time, seemingly after we had the gas fire apparently disconnected in the lounge, and an electric flame-effect one fitted instead. It's just as well none of us smoked, because the flames may not have been just effects.

We had the roof re-slated a few years ago. This too was interesting, as the roofers stripped all the slates from the roof, then disappeared for two weeks, by which time I had resorted to making phone calls from work because they were recorded, to insist that they came back. Fortunately they did, and so far we haven't leaked.

I'm not sure how we did all we did in the mid to late 2000s, though many families must know this feeling. Carole and I were working nearly 100 hours a week between us, and the lads ended up helping out. One Boxing Day, Max and I dug Carole's car out of the ice she had got stuck in on a visit in her role as Community Neo-Natal Nurse. On another Boxing Day some years before, when Carole was also working, I had taken all three lads on my house visits so they weren't home alone. They were very patient as they waited in the car, playing on whatever digital gadgets they had.

Over the years these gadgets were a mixed blessing, as they kept the lads interested and entertained, but we did have the occasional embarrassment. One afternoon in Tesco Tom and Adam, at the time in their mid teens, persuaded me to buy them GTA Vice City. I wasn't quite sure what this involved, but I should have guessed. Max was also with us, but seeing it was rated '18', sadly said, 'I can't play with that, can I, Dad?'

I replied, 'Well, okay, Max, so long as you don't go with any prostitutes,' just in time to hear 'Hello Dr Barker', from one of our patients passing with her trolley who had definitely heard the latter part of our conversation!

All our lads have been, and still are, very tolerant of my un-coolness, even though inside they must have been cringing at times. I didn't get to pick them up from school often, much to their relief, though I can still picture Max's expression when, walking down Southport Road one day, he realised the idiot who had a 10-foot tree sticking out of his car sunroof after visiting the garden centre was me.

He was way ahead of me even years before, though. While being driven home he decided he wasn't going to do what I wanted him to do when we got there.

'Max,' I said, mock firmly, 'one day you'll be driving your eleven-year-old son or daughter home from school, who won't do what you want him or her to do, and I'll be sat in the back saying, "Revenge is mine!"'

'No you won't, Dad,' replied Max promptly, 'because I'll have put you in a home!'

Tom decided that he wanted to study medicine at university, and we went to look at various medical schools. As usual, I got us lost, but I'm never too embarrassed to ask for directions.

In fact there were certain similarities in our predicament to a scene I can identify with in the 1994 film *Dumb and Dumber*. The character Jim Carrey plays is a limo driver, but he tries to impress an attractive young lady standing at a bus stop by asking her, from the back of the limo, for directions to the medical school where he says he is due to give a lecture.

The young lady replies in an obvious mid-European accent,

giving him directions.

Carrey's character in a roundabout way asks where she is from, and she replies, 'Austria'.

Carrey exclaims, 'Austria, well, g'day mate, let's throw another shrimp on the barbie.'

The young lady looks at him scornfully, the way young women sometimes looked at me years ago when I asked them out, and says, 'No, let's not.'

Tom didn't get into medical school at the first attempt so put the time to good use, got in at the second attempt and spent the remaining months on a gap year. He clearly matured during this experience, and also came back to say to Adam and Max that if they did not take a gap year he would slap them.

14. Work–Life Imbalance.

After 20 years as a GP partner I was still enjoying work, though there was rather a lot of it. Some of this was probably my doing, in the way I practised. I have been lucky to work with caring and compassionate colleagues throughout my career. We tried to go the 'extra mile' if needed to help people. For example, we still performed more home visits than the average practice. If people would really struggle to get to the surgery, either because of their medical conditions or logistical constraints such as a socially isolated single parent with several small children, one of whom was ill, we would visit. If someone's medical condition meant they could physically get to the surgery, but they genuinely had no funds or transport, I did sometimes pay for a taxi, and on rare occasions their prescription if they were not exempt, though I'm not sure that is strictly allowed.

Several times we GPs would end the day visiting, and when on call for Chorley Medics, on a visit in the middle of a dry night with a full moon in early June, I recall a previously worried mum with a poorly 19-month-old girl and no visible transport at home waving goodbye to us, and we all felt we were helping.

The patient and family contacts were enjoyable. Some of the computer documentation less so. I tried to data input appropriately, but sometimes I couldn't get the appropriate code recognised by my computer, probably due to my own inadequacies, and whereas some common conditions, symptoms, or examination findings didn't fit the data input box, some weird ones did.

One day I saw a lady who had painful feet after running the Paris marathon, not surprisingly. I tried to enter 'running', and while there was no 'running injury' or similar, the first choice was 'nose running' and the next 'accident involving cable car not running on rails – not otherwise specified'.

The following are all real examples of coding.

- T5407 'Hit by aircraft – parachutist injured'.
- T412 'Crushed by lifeboat after abandoning ship'.
- E221 'Bestiality (zoophilia).
- Eu65Y 'Necrophilia'.
- B9160 'Neoplasm of uncertain behaviour of the penis'.

When I tried to enter space-occupying lesion (SOL), for example due to a mass in the brain, the first computer default was to 'space craft'!

I still tried to be as conscientious and thorough as ever, though possibly still tending to the obsessional, and towards the end of each week I was pretty tired.

On two consecutive evenings, a Thursday then a Friday, I had requests for visits after surgery to see patients who may have needed compulsorily admitting to hospital under a Mental Health Act Section.

On the Thursday evening I spent two hours at a patient's house, the second actually with the patient, because for the first hour she had left the house. The psychiatrist and approved social worker also present decided they could not recommend a MHA section, though two previous psychiatrists had suggested this may be in the patient's best interest.

On the Friday I was asked to assess an elderly lady, who through mental illness seemed to be a danger to herself and possibly others. I visited as quickly as I could. When I got there I introduced myself but forgot to clarify who else was present. The patient herself was not. The gentleman there was our patient's husband, and I thought the other lady was the approved social worker whose assessment was also needed. I sat down next to her and chatted to the husband, who himself was understandably worried and couldn't really describe what had happened. Then the lady next to me said, 'My brother has taken her to the hospital.' She was the couple's daughter, and not the approved social worker, who had also gone.

Perhaps not very professionally I just rested my head on the daughter's shoulder, sighed, and said, 'Sorry, it's been a long week'.

At that time I started drinking alcohol probably too readily in the evenings after work, so then I tried to avoid drinking on weekday nights, usually successfully. It is easy to see how it becomes an unhealthy habit. I didn't have much time to exercise, and my weight ballooned up to just over 14 stones, my heaviest ever.

After a Thursday night working for Chorley Medics, hence little sleep for over 36 hours, I went to see the Australian Pink Floyd at the Guildhall in Preston, driven by my friend Danny, meeting there the lads' music teacher Jon, and his mum who is a Pink Floyd fan and had recently had her knee replaced.

After at least a couple of pints of lager, I was well away, and on leaving our seats after the show I stumbled into Jon's mum who, along with her crutches, went flying. Fortunately no harm was done and I phoned apologising profusely the next morning.

I decided to do something about my health, and started running again.

Adam had recently kindly bought me a page-a-day runners' calendar, and I pinched a couple of the quotes and had them printed on my running shirt. On the front was: 'This isn't sweat, it's my fat cells crying!' On the back: 'If you can read this, I'm not last!', which drew some sarcastic comments of 'Thanks very much, mate' on the rare occasions I overtook someone. There wasn't enough room for another one which may have been appropriate for the back: 'If found on ground please drag over finish line!'

I dieted, continued playing tennis with the lads, and in 2009 ran the London marathon with Adam, three weeks after his 18th birthday, raising funds for the Motor Neurone Disease Association.

I was 49 years old when I started training for this and was

getting various aches and pains I hadn't experienced before, particularly in my left leg. I went to see a physiotherapist who observed me running on the treadmill and asked her podiatry colleague for advice. After I clambered down from the treadmill, expecting compliments on my amazing physique and technique, the podiatrist said, 'Are you sure, running like that, you're only having problems with your leg?'! She kindly supplied me with custom-made orthotics, about which I am very enthusiastic, as they cured that problem.

Adam had become increasingly fit in his later school years and then at Runshaw College, and has subsequently kindly advised me on various aspects of my health, particularly musculoskeletal. After his gap year, during which he met his long-term girlfriend Liv, now fiancée, in Sydney, he went on to study physiotherapy at Nottingham University.

Being healthier physically certainly helps one function better mentally and intellectually. I continued to keep up to date and read around subjects of interest and also more widely, particularly in the *British Medical Journal* which I still think is a good read. Reading journals published internationally both in print and digitally does make one realise how fortunate we are in this country. A *BMJ* theme on world poverty had, in the same edition, an article regarding George Bush, who was making obtaining contraception worldwide more difficult.

When I did get too serious, or started expressing opinions or suggesting solutions to problems I was not qualified to comment on, my wonderful family kept me grounded, and still do. My in-laws that year bought me a card which said: 'It is better to be silent and thought a fool, than to speak out and remove all doubt'!

Carole continued to work very hard organising and carrying out the care of tiny babies in the community, as team leader. She did have bouts of supraventricular tachycardia (SVT) where her heart rate would suddenly flip into an abnormal rhythm of over 200 beats per minute, making her acutely unwell. She stoically bore these, and sometimes they stopped spontaneously, and on other occasions we went to A&E where she was given an intravenous drug to stop them. On two occasions we went to Wythenshawe hospital where cardiologists attempted to ablate the abnormal electrical pathways in her heart that were causing these.

Having spent an anxious day walking round Wythenshawe hospital car park while Carole underwent the second, and at the time unsuccessful, ablation, I went to work next morning, leaving her on her own. She had bravely tolerated the procedure, in significant pain while conscious.

During morning surgery I received a distressed call from Carole, who felt acutely unwell and disorientated. My colleagues kindly covered my work while I rushed home to see her and we spent the day on the medical assessment unit. Fortunately, no serious complications were identified, but I should never have left her alone.

I have tried to be a good husband, but writing this now makes me realise I could have done much better.

15. How to Be a Good Patient.

Working in a supportive group practice did mean that if unforeseen events suddenly cropped up, we could cover each other. On one occasion I respectfully asked one of our younger female partners to go home as she wasn't feeling well, and a week later she was on a ventilator with pneumonia! Fortunately she made a complete recovery. Most healthcare professionals battle on if feeling unwell, which is unwise, I found out some years later. We are not very good patients.

Over the years, as well as considering what makes a good doctor, I have thought about producing an informal and light-hearted guide to what makes a good patient. I do not intend to trivialise more serious illness, or cause offense.

Most of our Chorley patients are indeed patient. We worked flat out, and my colleagues still do, but with all that is currently expected in general medical practice, there are not enough resources to meet demand.

To be a really helpful patient, try not to become ill, or indeed consult at all if possible.

If you have to attend, try to have a clear idea why you are coming, and to have only one thing wrong with you.

Please try to present with typical symptoms so diagnosis is easy. This is of course often impossible, and one of the reasons general medical practice is fascinating.

The most dispiriting way consultations can start is with a big sigh; from the patient, that is.

I'd rather someone was agitated, or crying, as we could get

more quickly to helping.

Please let us know what is really troubling you, so we can address your concerns. In my days as a GP trainer we used to video-record consultations, with patients' consent of course, then earnestly discuss learning points with other GP trainers.

Consultations were 'mapped', and often both the patient and my trains of thought were all over the place. At times I thought, 'Am I making sense?', and occasionally I would think, 'Wow, I'm really bullshitting here!'

If you don't agree with a diagnosis, if one is made, or are not keen on a treatment recommended, please say so.

This was even more important on the thankfully rare occasions when prescribing errors were made, more often in the early days of computer prescriptions when a product was often defaulted to. On one occasion I intended to prescribe Pred Forte eye drops but instead prescribed Predfoam enemas. One of my partners prescribed support stockings '1 pair' (abbreviated to 'PR'). The computer interpreted this as 'to be taken PR' – per rectum. Our patient wondered why he was being instructed to insert his support stockings up his bottom.

My top tips to stay well are:

- Don't smoke.

- Drink alcohol in moderation only, or not at all

- Exercise regularly if possible.

- Don't eat too much fat or carbohydrates

- Try to take note of your family history. If there is a strong family history of, for example, breast or bowel cancer, or premature heart disease or diabetes, ask a healthcare professional for advice.

- Watch out for blood in your urine, bowel motions or sputum, and report it if you do notice any.

☐ Report any significant unintended weight loss, or significant weight gain.

☐ Report any lumps or swellings you have developed, no matter how embarrassing you may think they are.

16. Catching Diabetes.

In 2010 I started feeling tired again, and this time increasingly thirsty, so on 10 August, in between patients, I went for a wee and dipped it with a testing strip, which immediately turned dark blue on the glucose detector. At the end of surgery I tested my own capillary blood glucose and it was 17.1 millimoles per litre, normal random glucose being less than 11. I had a venous blood sample taken by our ever helpful practice nurses, which confirmed I had Type 2 diabetes. My first thought was that diabetes can take years off one's life expectancy, my second thought that there are worse things to have, so I will get on and behave myself and take treatment if needed, which it was.

I have never actually had a colonic irrigation, but I would imagine that the effects of starting the medication Metformin are similar. On a couple of occasions I almost had to say in surgery to patients, 'Well, I think we can help you, but before I do, please could you excuse me as I think I am about to s**t myself!'

One of my partners suggested that I had worked with diabetics so long, I'd caught it. I also recall one of our friends who is a diabetes specialist nurse asking her consultant what was the most important thing about diabetics he had learned in the 30 years before he retired. He replied, 'They do your f***ing head in!' And now I was one. Luckily for me it was easily controllable, though Carole rightly points out now that I might not need to be on three different diabetic medications if I didn't sneak 'Frank's diabetic ice cream', or the occasional (honest) chocolate.

I don't think my diabetes affected my work or vice versa. I also had my recurrently dislocating left shoulder fixed that year by an excellent colleague who did something like 700 shoulder procedures a year. I am not sure I could focus on one or two areas of the body for my whole career. One of my partners with experience in orthopaedics suggested that an holistic orthopaedic surgeon is one who cares for the whole bone. My surgeon was more than that. I can see why some medics decide to go into surgery, hopefully sorting something out, 'curing' it, though of course this is not always possible.

Working days got longer. I was usually in surgery before 6am going through lab results, letters, prescriptions, and tasks. We had an electronic 'workflow', which I likened to shovelling snow while it was still snowing. In the early hours I'd often see the milkman, the local baker, and colleagues in emergency services around. I felt rather like I was in Postman Pat's Greendale, or Trumpton.

Only I don't recall any episodes in those programmes where in one day I was asked to help, by the patient themselves, a relative, or a healthcare professional, six patients who said they were going to commit suicide.

None of them actually did at that time, though trying to help everyone given the lack of time and other resources, such as mental health workers, can be daunting.

Trying to save lives in general practice is not as dramatic, usually, as in secondary care, and the results of one's work take longer to become apparent. In one month, among other less significant diagnoses, I identified an early colon cancer, and an early testicular cancer, in patients who went on to do very well. Deciding, with the patient, if and when to refer to secondary care is one of the challenges of general practice, and a balance has to be struck between over and under investigating or treating.

Around this time a young lady with a complex medical history died, and I was asked to attend the Coroner's inquest. An open verdict was arrived at. I am sorry that sometimes even with our best efforts tragedies happen, and I still reflect on such people and wonder if anything could have been done differently.

'Significant event' meetings are held by primary healthcare teams, and sometimes more widely with secondary care, to see if lessons can be learned on an individual, multi-disciplinary team, or organisational basis.

17. Fast, Slow and In Between.

During 2011, partly thanks to some broadminded prescribing by her cardiologist, Carole's SVT heart rhythms had settled, but now I started getting episodes of sudden onset rapid regular heart rhythms, though not as fast as Carole's. I also had two episodes of atrial fibrillation (AF), a fast irregular rhythm. The cardiologist kindly saw me too, and fortunately couldn't detect any underlying heart disease, and from then on I took a 'pill in the pocket', Flecainide. This is an accepted way of trying to abort an abnormal heart rhythm when they occur, and it worked well for me. I still went running, and that year completed the Liverpool marathon.

I also really enjoyed taking part in Lakeland trails (www.lake-landtrails.org), runs of around 15km in beautiful Lake District scenery. My favourite is the Kentmere trail, starting and finishing in Staveley. There are two main events; the Challenge, for less competitive runners and faster walkers, and the Race. Needless to say I went in for the challenge. The dad of Tom's girlfriend (now wife) Jo did the race, about an hour faster than me. Still, on coming down from the last fell in glorious May sunshine in 2012 I felt I could fly.

In sharp contrast my dad's mobility had rapidly deteriorated in the preceding months, and in that year he started using a rollator, then a frame. Within a year he couldn't walk, and moved to live a mile from us in a retirement village with assisted living, in a wheelchair. I went with him to see neurologists, orthopaedic surgeons, and spinal surgeons. He has widespread spinal stenosis, where the spinal cord is compressed by a severely arthritic spine, and advanced arthritis of the hips and knees. There was no operative solution. At one time we thought he may have motor neurone disease, or even post-polio syndrome, having been unwell for several months as a child with an undefined illness, but investigations didn't confirm these.

After two years of scans and neurophysiology input, the spinal surgeon said to him, 'Well, you're knackered.' Dad took this pretty well, having always been practical and stoical. Without any self-pity he said to me, 'With Mum gone, I don't mind what happens.' Carole and her sister Joanne were hugely helpful and supportive during this time, and still are. Alec and Guy also do their best supporting us from Seattle, coming over when they can.

After what I had thought in previous years was reasonable work by our then practice manager, it became apparent that all was not well and that professional relationships were strained to say the least. To my shame I had been unaware of this, partly because I was so busy, and partly because I am sometimes oblivious to what is going on, which is not a good quality for a GP. Several very stressful months for many of the team followed, at the end of which we appointed a new practice business manager, who is excellent.

So relieved was I to have matters running relatively smoothly again, I was quite upbeat and grateful. In fact at a practice business meeting, one of my partners, Kevin, asked, 'Clive, if someone punched you in the face, would you thank them for it?', to which another partner, John, replied for me, 'Well, yes. It's better than a punch in the nuts!'

Surgery work was full-on as ever, my communications skills still suspect at times. I recall one lady attending concerned about a possible breast condition. She declined a chaperone, then starting the examination as always by inspection (i.e. looking), I heard myself say, 'looks good'. What I should have said perhaps was 'looks healthy'. On another occasion a man consulted with erectile dysfunction. As part of the history, and before examining him, I asked if he had any signs of swellings in his genitals, to which he replied, 'No, but I wish there were!' Another patient had erectile dysfunction which had been successfully treated with Sildenafil (Viagra). At that time certain criteria had to be fulfilled for this to be prescribed on an NHS prescription. He was borderline, but said, 'If I don't get my Viagra, doc, I'm f***ed,' to which I replied, 'Or not as the case may be.'

Visits were interesting too, with more people living longer, more diagnoses of dementia, and increasing numbers of residents in specialist dementia care homes.

At one of these I was trying to concentrate on one patient, when an elderly lady shouted at an even more elderly lady, 'You'd shag anyone, you would!' Disinhibition and agitation in dementia can be challenging to manage, raising safeguarding issues.

Deprivation of Liberty Safeguarding orders (DOLS) are sometimes used now to protect people who have lost capacity to be safe outside their environment so they don't leave on their own.

18. Wishing I Had as Much Sense as Our Lads...

In 2013 Tom and Adam both graduated very successfully. Their graduations were great fun in Liverpool and Nottingham respectively.

After Tom's, I put his graduation qualification documents down somewhere after he had asked me to look after them, to get a better photograph, and lost them! Tom was very mature about this and I was furious with myself. Fortunately in this digital age replacements are available for a small fee.

We enjoyed meeting our sons' friends and their friends' families. For all my outwardly confident manner I do get quite nervous making a lot of new acquaintances and introduced myself to one of Adam's friend's families initially as 'Adam's mum', and then as 'Carole's mum'! This was *before* I'd had a drink.

In the following months Max and I did an England-wide tour of six universities, from Newcastle in the north to Southampton in the south. I knew nothing about media, culture, and communications, so found it fascinating. Initially Max seemed quite reserved on these visits, though he was clearly inspired by the universities, saying in one grand building, 'Hey, I feel cleverer already.' By the time we got to the sixth and final open day, when a prospective tutor asked, 'Who is coming here to university to try and get as far away as possible from their parents?', his hand shot up. Since then Max has also achieved a high level of success and is working in marketing communications.

At Max's graduation, apparently Newcastle graduates weren't allowed to rent mortar boards because in previous years too many had ended up in the Tyne (the mortar boards that is, not the graduates, I think).

Seeing all these bright, enthusiastic, and fun young people really gives us hope for the future.

I had said to one of Tom's peers, soon to be his best man, that they had all obviously worked hard and played hard. Matthew replied, 'Yes we have, but not necessarily in that order.'

When our 'boys' come home, hearing the banter between them is hilarious. Like any youngsters they have had their moments of, shall we say, disagreement, but they're all mates now and it's good to see them supporting each other. Although I am often still acutely embarrassing, they are very tolerant of me. I give advice, even when it's not been asked for and not needed.

Tom once summed that up: 'Dad, you don't half chat some s**t, but occasionally you say something helpful.'

Going out with them can be eventful too. One Friday evening in 2013, we went out to celebrate our Australian niece's 18th birthday as she was visiting. Afterwards, Adam and Liv and our niece Maxine invited Carole and I into Chorley to 'Spoons' – Wetherspoons. Carole was driving and therefore sober, and I was not. On that occasion Max had gone home with Carole's sister Joanne in another car.

Adam and Liv kindly bought me a Jägerbomb – Jägermeister and highly caffeinated Red Bull, I understand. I had heard of those, but to me it tasted like one of my childhood soft drinks, dandelion and burdock, so I had another.

We got back home to find Max waiting up and chastising us, 'Where have you been?' I went to bed after reading for a while, expecting to feel the effects of this unwise imbibing, but nothing happened, until 6am. Then I woke up with a start, sat bolt upright, sweating profusely, wanting to vomit, and with a heart rate that seemed totally out of control.

I stumbled around the house, desperately looking for my 'pills in the pocket', along with anti-emetics to stop me vomiting, and painkillers for my exploding head. Then I passed out for another four hours, after which I gradually awoke, wondering if I should put this learning experience in my next appraisal.

We have enjoyed getting to know the lads' girlfriends' families too. After feeling rather weedy hearing that Tom's Jo's dad was a firefighter who once ran a marathon in around two and a half hours, I tried to impress Liv's parents. During a fun first weekend with them, after a hospitable evening, at breakfast I asked with interest, 'What's that interesting tree in your garden, with bulbous red things at the end of the branches, that look like apples?' They patiently replied, 'It's an apple tree.'

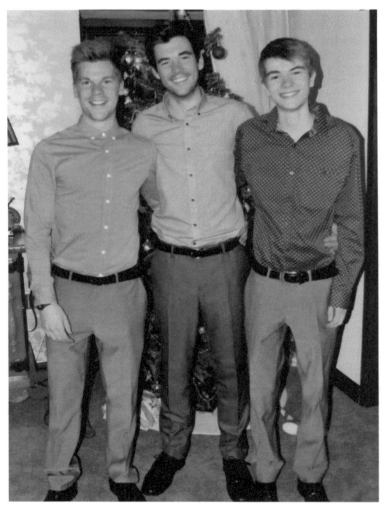

Our lads from left to right, Adam, Tom, Max,
Christmas 2011

19. Friends and Families.

Doctors do tend to moan a lot. In the years of Primary Care Trusts, the medical profession, including myself, had implied that we didn't need all these managers to tell us what to do; doctors could do it more efficiently. So, at just the time that spending on the NHS in real terms stopped increasing, Andrew Lansley, the then Secretary of State for Health, effectively said, 'Okay, you do it.'

Clinical Commissioning Groups, created in the Health and Social Care Act of 2012, replaced PCTs on 1 April 2013. These CCGs were set up to manage up to 80% of the NHS's £100 billion plus annual budget. GPs, with the support of colleagues, some of whom were made redundant from the PCTs then re-employed by CCGs, are trying to organise and commission care from various providers of services, with a limited budget. Some of my local GP colleagues work very hard trying to balance being a practising GP with work for the CCG. How they do this, I really don't know. Our friend Dinesh managed this for many years, though he always has been much better at multi-tasking than people like me. In fact, in what little spare time he has, he does things such as fix his children's smartphones, looking up how to do it on YouTube. In comparison, I have severe learning difficulties.

Around this time, Jane, our senior partner for the last six years, retired. She had been hugely supportive all my time in the partnership, and very wise.

I therefore became Senior Partner, though I usually referred to myself as the oldest partner.

I felt rather like my brother Guy, who in his case modestly says, 'I got where I am today by a succession of people in positions of authority mistaking my enthusiasm for competence.'

As well as being 'responsible clinician for complaints', I continued in my role as GP diabetes lead, though in reality our excellent practice nurses managed this.

I also took part in child health surveillance clinics (baby clinics), which often left me with a headache trying to remember to check everything I was supposed to while the little ones often bawled through the clinic. My mind was so boggled by the time I was examining the last baby one day, that when I explained to the parents that I was going to check her hips, Mum and Dad looked rather concerned, as the baby in question was lying there completely naked, with an impressively sized penis and scrotum on show.

Another role I had was 'substance misuse co-lead' in the practice, trying to manage those with illicit drug misuse, with the guidance of a specialist team in the community.

I was also the medical representative in our monthly multidisciplinary team meetings, where team members would get together and make sure our organisation was functioning well, and act on any feedback we'd received from colleagues or patients. We usually did quite well in the 'friends and family feedback', where patients were asked if they would recommend our practice to friends or family. Usually over 90% of respondents said they would, though at times we would receive demoralising comments expanding on why they wouldn't recommend us, such as 'sh*t' and 'the waiting room is full of sick people'.

My business sense has never been very objective and on a number of occasions I felt I needed to apologise to my partners for my weaknesses.

GPs are allowed to charge for non-NHS services, such as completing travel insurance claims. Our practice has always charged at the lower end of the recommended rate advised by the BMA and Local Medical Committee, but I found it hard to charge someone I'd got to know well over 30 years for a travel insurance report after a holiday had to be cancelled due to one of the prospective travellers or a family member dying. Admittedly, these monies could have been re-invested into patient care.

Many patients have become friends over the years. A wonderful lady who lived on the same road as we did in our first house developed a brain tumour. She was a remarkable lady, positive right up to the end. On the day she died I visited her again to confirm her life was over, then headed back to the baby clinic (child health surveillance clinic) and hoped it wasn't too obvious that the crying babies were being seen by a GP who himself had just been crying.

I have also learned a lot from patients, including the phrase 'the price you pay for love is grief'. This was a lady in her eighties, who had visited me with her husband previously. He had subsequently died with a lymphoma. They were inseparable, having a shared love for a vintage car they used to drive to shows in. They also made a mean sloe gin, a bottle of which I was pleased to receive each year.

Another moving family relationship which I was privileged to learn about was between a lovely lady and her father, who was undergoing ultimately unsuccessful treatment for a malignancy. As they waited at the hospital for another cycle of his treatment, our patient was understandably feeling low and upset that her father was going through this. As he was about to undergo treatment he asked her to visit the paediatric oncology department of the hospital, which helped her to put things in perspective.

Although working out of hours, particularly at night, had been for me a quintessential part of being a family doctor, shortly before I became Senior Partner I decided to stop working nights.

One Thursday night, after getting my head down on the bed at Chorley Medics base for about 10 minutes and falling into a fitful sleep, the phone went at about 4am. A home visit was being requested. I found myself thinking, in a dazed semi-awake fugue-like state, 'How can I get out of going?' That was literally a wake-up call. I went on the visit, saw the patient, and the next day gave notice that I would not be working for Chorley Medics again. The time you realise that, for whatever reason, you may not be able to put yourself in a position to make a diagnosis, then that is the time to quit.

20. A Way of Medicine and Life.

By 2015, at the age of 56, I was rushing around so much it was unhealthy; 'run ragged' as Carole put it. Work was mad busy, and I was at Library House surgery well over 60 hours a week. I was sneaking in at weekends before or after visiting Dad or going to Tesco, walking Molly, or even going for a run. Carole was understandably worried what this was doing to me and us, as was I.

On one occasion I went shopping in Chorley, and while I was there I went into work to do some catch-up administration. Carole thought it would be nice to meet and have a coffee, so phoned me once she'd arrived in town.

'Where are you now?' she enquired.

'Er, I'm outside the sports shop on Market Street,' I bluffed.

'Well, that's strange,' she replied, 'because I'm outside your surgery window, and I'm sure I can see someone who looks very like you in there.'

Oops!

Some mornings I would get up before 4am to go to work, coming home after seven in the evening. There is a lot of work in general medical practice other than consulting, though the long hours were in part my own fault, through not being very efficient and forever 'safety netting'.

By Friday evenings I was done in. On one occasion visiting a dementia care home to see a patient on a late visit I walked into the wardrobe instead of the bathroom to wash my hands.

Although I worked long hours, at least in my job I could come home most nights to the support of my family. I wasn't away for days or weeks on business, or on an oil rig in the North Sea. I wasn't sharing quarters with men who were snoring and farting all night long, and I haven't spent up to eight months without going home, like the crew on a cruise ship looking after lucky people like us.

Outside of work I wasn't much help to Carole looking after our home. I did go to see Dad in his retirement village regularly, and had unexpected nocturnal visits to Library House when the burglar alarm went off, as I was now first on the contact list, only to learn later that spiders in the sensors were usually the problem.

Some years before, Dad had kindly gifted the premises of the dental practice he'd built up over 35 years, which had also been our home from 1964-1973, to Alec and Guy's families and mine, and we rent it to a dental company. I was also involved in managing this.

Sadly, by 2015, Dad's cognitive abilities were deteriorating. His GPs have kindly seen him and more recently he has been assessed when in hospital, and although he is taking appropriate treatment, he remains very forgetful.

He is very philosophical, and accepting of the situation, as always. Three years earlier when Guy, after discussion with us, said to Dad that we didn't think he should drive, Dad replied, 'Oh, okay then,' and never did again. More recently when one of his sisters, my aunt, became unwell after an infection, I asked him not to worry if she phoned sounding confused, he said, 'Oh, another one of us'! Fortunately my aunt made a good recovery.

As Mum had suggested when she was ill, and indeed before that, we should live life to the full and 'go for it', Alec, Guy and I journeyed on a fascinating cruise down the river Nile with Dad in 2007. Alec and Guy returned to their homes in Seattle afterwards, and saying goodbye to Dad seemed to age him 10 years, making me realise how tough it must be to say goodbye to loved ones living far away round the world, but how special it is when they get together. Within hours Dad was back to his normal chirpy self.

Not long after that Dad and I travelled to Tasmania to see the family of Maurice, the medical officer in Cyprus in the mid to late

1950s when Dad was the dental officer and they were doing their National Service. Maurice himself had died some years before of lung cancer, though he had never smoked, but his wife Noreen and their family have kept in touch over the decades. I think Mum would be proud of us.

At the time of writing Dad has recently celebrated his 85th birthday, and no Barker has made it to 85 before, so at least he is still with us, not distressed, and able to have some fun with us at this time.

The last time Dad was able to use his computer was after I had proudly shown him Tom's CV, though neither Tom nor I had realised he had headed the document 'Cirriculum Vitae'. I visited Dad shortly after to see half a dozen attempts to print the phrase spelt correctly, which he had, Curriculum Vitae.

On a Friday in 2015 I took Dad to his 60th year university reunion; he'd graduated in 1955. About 14 of the original year of 36 was able to make it, and it was moving to hear them singing 'We'll meet again', though this was their last formal reunion.

That Sunday I ran the Liverpool Rock and Roll Marathon in 4 hours and 51 minutes. Buoyed up by music, usually from live bands, every mile, I was urged on by songs such as 'Born to Run', 'These Boots Are Made for Walking', and 'Penny Lane'.

The night before, I stayed in a local hotel and took myself out to an Italian restaurant and ate lots of pasta, accompanied by a bottle of white wine, partly because this seemed to make more economic sense than buying it by the glass. When the waitress found out I was running the marathon the next day she said, 'I like your style'. Seeing the photographs of me crossing the finish line the next day, 'style' is not one of the words anyone would apply to my look. If ever there is an Olympic event called 'the long distance run for people who have had too much to drink the previous evening', I'm in with a good chance of a medal.

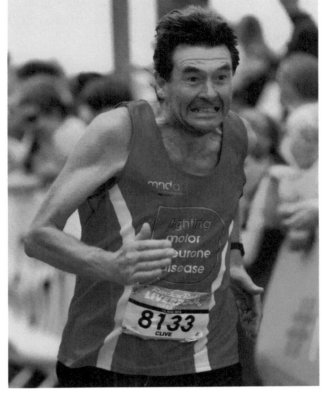

My 'style' finishing Liverpool Marathon 2015 (about which my brother also pointed out I'd missed 'arm day' at the gym!)

Some of my training consists of running to collect the car from restaurant car parks, in the days after going out for meals and getting taxis home.

I am running the 2019 London Marathon, with Tom and Adam, in support of the Motor Neurone Disease Association at the age of 60, and I am going to take it a lot more seriously.

Carole and I always try to touch base with our lads at least by phoning on a Sunday. Neither of us are on Facebook, though Carole has a smartphone and regularly communicates with them in some digital form or another.

My brothers, Alec and Guy, Carole's sister Joanne, and my

secretaries would update us regarding posts on social media. Alec summed up the two most frequent subjects involving the lads as 'Manchester United, and beautiful women'!

Several years before, we held a family reunion, the lead organiser being Frances, one of my cousins. Every descendent of my grandparents Jack and Doris, through Dad and his three sisters , was there with their families. Frances was a shining example of how to live life to the full, right up until the day she died in 2015 at the age of 48 from cancer. She and her husband Nick had a break from the hospital on Valentine's Day to see the film *Brief Encounter*, three days before Frances died.

I cried quietly during the first part of the service to celebrate her life, then their children Ana and Alex stood up and read *The Owl and the Pussycat*, and then Nick read his tribute, and these really were a celebration.

Frances' nephew Will and some friends played 'Mr Blue Sky' live. Frances certainly had danced in the rain rather than waiting for the sun.

Following the service I had too much to drink and, taking the train from London, almost missed getting off at Preston station, which would have meant waking up in Glasgow.

Most of our generation in both Carole's family and mine have luckily remained well, and we celebrate reunions when we can. Carole's brother Pete came over from Australia, and a surprise 54th birthday party one Friday evening was sprung on him. After a busy week I had fun on the Friday evening and the next morning photos of my 'dancing' were sent to Carole. This consisted of my shuffling from one foot to the other with my head back and my mouth open, for some reason alone on the dance floor. Pete said it was good to see me let my hair down. I told this to Guy not long after, to which he responded, 'Yes, you let your hair down, and your wife!'

I am aware while writing this, that chapters I intend to be mainly about work blur into life outside work, and chapters in which I intend to discuss life outside work develop into issues from my working life. I guess that this is because the two have been inexorably linked.

21. Teamwork.

In the run-up to the 2015 general election, as M.D. from *Private Eye* put it, 'rhetoric on the NHS has descended into a predictable fantasy-promises auction'– by most parties. The UK was bottom of the Group of 7 (G7) countries (who produce over half of the world's economic output), regarding funding of healthcare. The internal market created within the NHS cost around £4.5 billion a year, locums to fill positions left vacant by inadequate staffing levels cost over £2 billion a year, and still £640 million a year was spent on management consultants.

Morale wasn't helped when Secretary of State Jeremy Hunt suggested that worried doctors had 'no sense of vocation', criticising doctors and the BMA for not wanting to work even more at weekends. Ironically, I was reading this electronically at work one Sunday morning while two of my partners were seeing patients in surgeries.

No one locally was asking me to put these hours in, but in trying to be as thorough as I could be, and meet what I thought were others' expectations, I didn't let up. I recall lying in my dentist's chair having a filling replaced, actually enjoying the experience as it was the most relaxing half hour I'd had for a while.

My neck and lower back were painful due to radiologically confirmed degenerative changes. I was getting muscle contraction headaches and severe heartburn. I went for an upper gastrointestinal endoscopy which showed gastritis (inflammation of the stomach), then went back to work within the hour, and was shortly after wolfing down sandwiches with one hand while data-inputting lab links with the other.

By the end of 2015 my working pattern was not healthy for either myself or my family life. I was too tired to be as aware as I wanted to be about what was going on in the world, and most importantly what our lads were up to. On three consecutive weekday evenings I fell asleep in the lounge, in the study, and on the toilet, by around 9pm.

After discussing matters with Carole, I asked my partners if I could work 'three-quarters' time from April 2016, with a view to retiring in March 2019, my 60th birthday month. They kindly agreed and Alex, the latest doctor in the practice, having trained with us at various levels, joined us permanently, much to everyone's relief.

The run-up to going three-quarters time was spent preparing for a Care Quality Commission inspection (CQC), which all GP practices had to have. In my previous patient newsletter I had asked patients that if they saw a group of earnest people studiously making notes, just in case they were the CQC visitors, please could they try to look healthy and happy.

The following paragraphs are excerpts from our Spring 2016 Newsletter, concluding with my personal explanation regarding what I was doing.

The most notable event so far this year has been our first inspection by the Care Quality Commission who monitor, inspect, and regulate health and social care services. Some of you may be aware of the work of the CQC, but briefly this is a very comprehensive examination of services provided, with information obtained from practice team members and patients, regarding whether our services are safe, effective, caring, responsive to people's needs, and well-led.

We are pleased to report that we were rated 'Good' in all these areas.

After the visit they analysed their findings and reported to the Chief Inspector of General Practice, who then summarised the findings in a letter:

☐ Patients said they were treated with compassion, dignity and respect and they were involved in their care and decisions about their treatment.

☐ The practice has good facilities and was well equipped to treat patients and meet their needs.

☐ Staff assessed patients' needs and delivered care in line with current evidence-based guidance. Staff had the skills, knowledge and experience to deliver effective care and treatment.

☐ There was an open and transparent approach to safety and an effective system in place for reporting and recording significant events.

☐ Risks to patients were assessed and well managed.

☐ Information about services and how to complain was available and easy to understand.

☐ There was a clear leadership structure and staff felt supported by management. The practice proactively sought feedback from staff and patients, which it acted on.

☐ The care was delivered from a family perspective with a dynamic team.

☐ The practice was working seven days a week to ensure continuity of care for its patients.

☐ There was a good supportive environment for staff with a positive atmosphere.

In April 2016, I am reducing my sessions worked at the practice to three-quarter time, having been full-time for 30 years. Although still as committed as ever to working for you, our patients, and our team here, at the age of nearly 57 I am finding I am increasingly tired at the end of the days and week, and I have a duty to all of you, and to the General Medical Council to make sure I am able and safe to continue practising to what I would like to think is a high standard. Although I am lucky with my health, and as some of you know and have kindly been supportive, I am still 'running', but do have a number of medical conditions myself now. On the reverse of race event numbers there are sections on which one has to enter medical conditions and medication taken, and I am finding there isn't enough space!

It doesn't seem 30 years since some of you were saying to me, in a well-meaning way, 'That's all very well Dr Barker, but I don't think Dr Platt would do it like that!' I am very lucky to have 7 excellent GP Partners and a very supportive team, and if you are unable to obtain an appointment with me, with my reduced hours, please could I respectfully request that you see one of my very able and more up to date colleagues. I am grateful to my partners and team and yourselves for your support in this, before I retire in 3 years' time.

I have written a lot about what I was doing, but it is important to point out that just about everyone else in our team was working to capacity too. Our dedicated team started well before 5am with our cleaners who also made my coffee and breakfast. The reception team got in often before 7am, the doctors and nurses not long after, along with our administration, management, prescribing, and secretarial teams. I would try and leave before 7pm, but many of the GPs, nurses, and others would leave later than this, going home in the dark by which time their young kids would be in bed.

Nationwide, primary healthcare teams are doing their absolute best, but there are not enough trained healthcare professionals to fulfil demand. I am acutely aware that, while my overall contribution was negligible in the grand scheme of things, reducing my hours didn't help that situation, but I hope readers understand why I had to.

22. Being Uncool.

My day away from surgery in the spring and summer 2016 was put to good use by Carole and I. We enjoyed some lovely walks together, though I got us lost almost every time. I've bought all sorts of guides and tried to match them with Ordnance Survey maps to hopeless effect.

I started doing long-postponed jobs such as clearing out the garage; inhaling large amounts of dust and particles from mice droppings. I'm hoping they don't manifest themselves in years to come as some odd lung disease.

For the last six years we have had a mad springer spaniel, Molly, and I could take her out more. Molly was bought in just the same way as Ruby, with me thinking that my days of taking our dog's faeces for a walk in a biodegradable bag were over. It was impossible though not to be affected by her crazy enthusiasm when we saw her at the kennels and these years when she has been part of our family have proved we were right to choose her.

Just when I thought I couldn't get any less cool, I exceeded my own expectations. On a lovely spring morning before setting off to London, not to collect our CBE from the Queen for Services to Medicine, which mysteriously still hasn't arrived, but to see Adam and Liv, I took Molly for a walk in Astley Park.

Trying to take a photograph of her beside the blossoming flowers and trees, with Astley Hall behind, I fell backwards into a bog. On getting back to the car I had to take my trousers off as they were caked in mud, and after putting them on the back seat of my car, I couldn't find my car keys. They were of course in one of the deep pockets of my muddied trousers. I knelt facing backwards on the driver's seat and fumbled around to find the keys, only for my bum, clad in muddy underpants, to press on the car horn on the steering wheel, which went off loudly, attracting the attention of nearby people. Whether they were my patients, or went to the police to report indecent exposure, or took themselves off for counselling, I still don't know.

When I got home I surprised Carole, and Mandy, our long-suffering house-cleaning friend, by starting to tell them about this, all while wearing the dog's towel.

Still, as someone who earlier that week bought a plastic Thunderbird 2 model from Tesco and superglued it to the dashboard to represent my car, Virgil, the big green Volvo (like big green Thunderbird 2), I was never going to be cool.

Molly cheers us up when the lads aren't around, apart from on the very rare occasions when I started the day at five in the morning by skating in her diarrhoea on the kitchen floor. On one occasion I had an SVT while clearing this up, and Molly, sensing I didn't feel well, tried to lick me better. Her enthusiasm is infectious, probably literally.

Another dog I was very fond of over the years was Snoopy, along with his friends. In one cartoon strip Charlie Brown (the wishy-washy character, strangely with the same initials as me) or one of the other kids walks past Snoopy saying, 'You must be crazy wearing a fur coat on a hot day like this!'

Snoopy thinks, 'I'd rather sacrifice comfort for style.'

In my case, I'd always prefer to sacrifice style for comfort, much to my family's disappointment.

When feeling well, which was most of the time, I was able to train more for runs, and was seen running in a park by a patient who commented that I'd said I was too tired to be a full-time GP partner now, but was still okay to run. It's a different kind of tiredness. When at work it's very much mental exertion; when running, it's physical.

On another occasion when I went running, two young men were sitting in Astley Park near the cenotaph smoking, and drinking what looked like rather strong lager, one of whom I recognised as one of our substance misuse patients. He greeted me by saying 'Y'right, Bolt?' To mistake me for Usain Bolt he must have been very high indeed.

That spring in the Liverpool half-marathon, at 10.5 miles I was feeling good when I tripped over a cobble as I ran down the Mersey River front, lacerating the left side of my forehead. The young St John's team were very helpful, bandaged me up, and I completed the half-marathon, getting a few more shouts of encouragement than usual.

Perhaps I should have gone straight to A&E instead of having lunch with Tom and his friends first, but as a diabetic on treatment who had just run a half-marathon, a lager shandy and burger was indicated.

Then I went to the A&E department, where a maxillo-facial doctor kindly sewed up my forehead, commenting, 'You're going to look rather like Harry Potter after this.' I didn't understand the significance at the time, but thought this probably wasn't a good thing to hear. I have a barely visible Y-shaped scar, rather than Harry Potter's lightning bolt.

Unfortunately, having a scar like a Y chromosome hasn't made me 'man up' much. Carole and I were able to go on date nights where we would go and see a film and sometimes have a meal in a nearby restaurant. Nowadays the meal has to be first, because on one occasion we went to the cinema first, saw *A Monster Calls* about a youngster whose mum is dying, and I was still crying in the restaurant. I'd say it might be the andropause, but since I cried 20 years ago at *The Lion King*, not much has changed.

On one of my walks with Carole we were overtaken by our friend and colleague, Danny, out on his visits with two medical students in tow. Naturally, I told them not to believe anything he said.

Danny had worked very hard to help set up a team who could tender to provide local services by and for local people, including musculoskeletal services and urgent care, within the NHS. Tendering for these and other services was open to Any Qualified Provider (AQP), including private companies.

Our practice had previously provided a good deep vein thrombosis (DVT) assessment service, though this has been recommissioned elsewhere, outside our control. Some of my partners wanted to provide services ourselves within the NHS, as it was thought we were a big enough practice to do so. Thus my loyalties were divided. I wanted to support bids of teams in groups of local GP practices, yet I also wanted to support my partners and our practice. As usual, I was trying to please everyone all of the time, which is of course impossible. In the end, I didn't please anyone, and I worry that this internal market is dividing doctors, colleagues, and friends.

23. Time to Go.

It was during 2016 that the people of the UK voted narrowly for Brexit. Carole and I couldn't believe it initially. I am aware my political and economic knowledge is scant, but I can't see how it can be wise to become less internationally involved and co-operative with our near neighbours, in the 21st century. Perhaps it is partly because I'm aware that the NHS has been kept going by overseas colleagues to a large extent for the last 50 or more years.

As for the lies that implied that £350 million a week would be spent on the NHS rather than Europe, words fail me. We are hardly appearing to be 'strong and stable' at present.

Still, at least we live in a country where ordinary citizens can vote, and the Government won't send in the army if the result goes against them, or another group attempts a violent coup.

As autumn drew on, it became clear that three-quarter time working wasn't working as I had envisaged, for me or for patients. Again, partly through my own doing, trying to help with continuity, it felt like I was trying to cram full-time working into three quarters of the hours, even with the support of my colleagues. I had managed to reduce my hours at the surgery to a little over 50 a week, but I felt more stressed again. Several of my brighter colleagues do some of their administration work electronically from home, but I felt that once I started working from home, I may never stop. Also, I was too dim to get the IT set-up, though Simon, our IT and Operations Manager, had infinite patience with me over the years. He even set me up with a standing work-station. This meant that when consulting with patients I would sit down, yet during the hours of administration time, the computer and small desk would effortlessly lift up. My back felt better within days, and I imagined I was Rick Wakeman (minus the long hair and silly hat) in the early 1970s prog-rock era, playing multi-layered keyboards – cool!

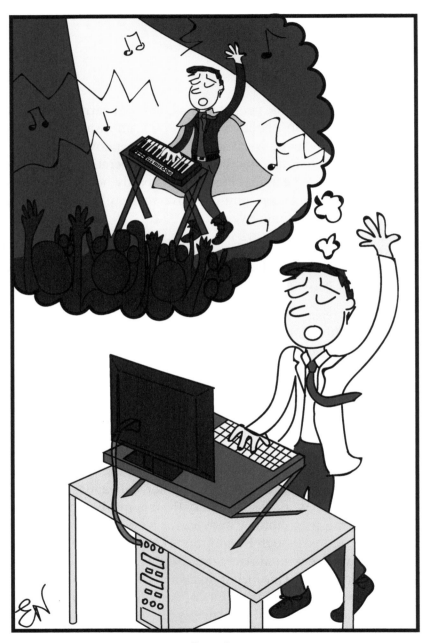

Prog-doc

If I hadn't been in on a Friday or sneaked in over the weekend, I would get up at four in the morning on a Monday to be in work before five, to study the avalanche into my inbox even though my colleagues kindly covered anything urgent on the days at the end of the week when I didn't (in theory) work. I slept badly on a Sunday night and felt guilty that perhaps I hadn't been as patient with Dad who I collected and brought round to us on a Sunday afternoon for tea, while Carole cooked for everyone who was around, including her dad and mum, now aged 94 and 84 respectively. My back would pull, lifting my dad in and out of Virgil, and on occasions we fell on top of each other. All this time he was doing his best, including apologising for 'not being as bright as I was' – heartbreaking again.

Carole and I would get away from time to time, and in October 2016, on a gloriously sunny autumn day, I ran the Munich half-marathon in 2 hours 13 minutes. Who'd have thought that 44 years after watching the 1972 Olympics as a scrawny, 13-year-old cross-country runner, I would be running into that very stadium. I almost cried when I saw the Olympic tower from 2km away, and not just because my muscles were aching so much.

Most patients and their families were wonderful, and I still loved the job, but there was also still too much of it.

The week beginning Monday, 12 December 2016 made me review my plans again during a period of reflection over Christmas and the New Year.

I was late getting back from the home visits that Monday morning, which I was writing up before trying to get to our weekly meeting which started at one o'clock. I had forgotten that one of the CCG Prescribing Team was coming to talk to us, though I was reminded by an 'instant message' on my screen. I rushed upstairs to the presentation, and gradually my heart sank. Although I had always tried to prescribe in line with current guidelines, and have never received any individualised negative feedback or adverse figures, our practice was prescribing above the national average both in amount and in certain types of antibiotics.

As most people will know, this is an increasingly worrying

global issue. I am aware that I may have been slower than some to reduce my antibiotic prescribing, and I do know that overall my partners
when appropriate tended to prescribe less often than they would have
in earlier times.

However, I would have difficulty, for example, on seeing a distressed young child with a high fever and clinically a throat and/or
ear infection, confidently explaining to his or her parent that this may
be viral and the majority will settle after two to three days, advising
only painkillers and treatment for the fever in the meantime. I would
of course discuss this strategy, but probably had a lower threshold for
prescribing a course of antibiotics, or giving a delayed prescription if
the symptoms didn't settle. Some of these would turn out to be bac-
terial infections requiring treatment later, though admittedly serious
complications through not prescribing antibiotics are rare.

Similarly, if a patient had symptoms and signs of a kidney infection, I would tend to prescribe an antibiotic that microbiologically
locally had a sensitivity rate (and therefore would usually be effective), of over 85% (for example a cephalosporin), rather than one with
a sensitivity rate of 75% (for example trimethoprim). This may seem
sensible for the individual patient, but may be less so for the community long-term, risking further development of resistance (to cephalo-
sporins) and, because it is a broader spectrum antibiotic, risking side
effects such as clostridium difficile, though that is rare in a seven-day
course.

Again, was I putting the needs of the individual before the
needs of the wider population?

I worried that I was becoming the proverbial dinosaur, and
holding my colleagues back.

In the middle of that week we received a letter from our MP.
A patient had written to him, rather than us, expressing concern about
the way a request one weekend for an urgent appointment for her baby
had been handled. Although opening seven days a week, our weekend resources were limited, and when all appointments had been filled
we respectfully requested that, in line with NHS guidance, our patient
contacted the usual out-of-hours service via 111, and they would be

seen by a local colleague.

The baby in question turned out to be fine, though we did understand how concerned her mum must have been, and we did try to address that, but then Mum said she was going to the NHS Ombudsman.

As the responsible clinical person for complaints, I tried to support all parties, and the complaint went no further.

The same week another patient was angry and upset that 'the hospital said the GPs were prescribing wrongly'. I looked into this, and confirmed we had not prescribed wrongly, and we never found out what the hospital had actually said.

At the end of my working week I was in early going through letters delivered to the surgery the previous evening, which I hadn't yet had chance to read.

One letter was from the relative of a patient who had a long-term medical condition. Although our patient was very stoical and seemed satisfied with the care given, the family member thought the medical care was inadequate and said that unless this improved a higher authority would become involved.

I thought I had done my best, and that I couldn't do any more, though perhaps with being three-quarter time my continuity could have been better, though I know my colleagues would have helped out if I'd not been there.

I can still recall standing at my desk in my room at 6am that December, pitch black and cold outside, putting the letter gently down and realising 'it's time to go'.

At no time has Carole put pressure on me to reduce my hours, or retire from the surgery, but I obviously discussed my plans with her and our lads. Max was home shortly afterwards for Christmas, and had been telling us one evening how his final year at uni and his dissertation were going, and to my shame I forgot some of what he had told us, my brain was so full and addled. Fortunately, he is very patient, and told me again the next evening.

In mid January at the monthly practice business meeting in the evening, I gave my partners and management team my letter of intention to retire from the practice at the end of August 2017. This was a little longer than the required six months' notice, but I felt it was the least I could do, after all their years of support for me, to hang on until the school summer holidays were over so they could take a well-deserved break. Earlier that day, a couple of hours after getting in, I had an SVT, which usually responded to my pill in the pocket, lying down flat on the floor, and taking some deep breaths. One of my partners, Rachel, was rather surprised on calling in to my room to find me so, leaving a message on a patient's answerphone. I hadn't had chance to phone all my partners the day before, but had spoken to Rachel, and to Suzanne, the next soon-to-be senior partner and also a huge support over the years.

I don't think my partners wanted to get rid of me, but they were all understanding and supportive of my decision. I had enjoyed being Senior Partner and every one of our team had been very helpful over the years. I'd tried to be there for all our team members, but as in other areas, I worried that at times I'd had difficulty reconciling the needs of each person with the needs of the practice as a whole. It has been pointed out to me that if individuals within an organisation are happy, then the organisation usually works well, and I hope this has been the case.

24. Chronic Common-Sense Deficiency Syndrome.

Over many years Ewan and Karen, my best man and Carole's bridesmaid (along with her sister Joanne), have been wonderfully hospitable in their lovely home in Pentraeth, Anglesey, overlooking Red Wharf Bay. In fact we bought them a visitor's book recently to try to record some of the many friends who come and go.

Before it became impractical, Dad and I were lucky enough to go to stay on a number of occasions, along with the wheelchair, a ramp, and 'Little Nelly'. This is a scooter that can be dismantled and put in the boot of Virgil, and is so easy to reassemble even I can do it. Ewan commented that it was the equivalent of James Bond's mini helicopter.

In recent years many friends have movingly helped Dad. Literally movingly in some cases, with Paul and Julie and my cousin Richard and his wife Pam kindly helping him move house. Our friend Dave who is a medical engineer has extended his skills and even fixed Dad's electric bed. Other friends and our extended family visit when they can.

In the lads' childhoods we would all go and visit Ewan and Karen, and their daughters Ellie and Hannah, then as the years went by and the younger generation had their own commitments we couldn't visit as much. After not seeing Ewan and Karen and the girls for a while, they visited us when the girls were in their mid teens, as were Tom and Adam. Adam thoughtfully commented about the two pretty young ladies, 'Hmmm, they've changed a bit, haven't they'. A long way from playing Big Bad Wolf in their garden.

On Sunday, 5 March 2017 Tom and I ran the Anglesey half-marathon. Rachel and her husband Angus also took part, finishing ahead of me, as did Tom; way ahead in fact.

I had a sore throat the day before, but thought nothing of it, and Tom and I carb-loaded on a delicious roast dinner, courtesy of Ewan and Karen, on the Saturday evening.

The weather was atrocious; cold and windy, with driving rain. I completed the run soaked to the skin and shivering.

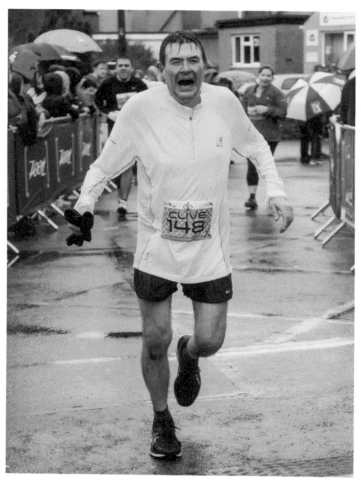

Me finishing the Anglesey Half Marathon March 2017, 10 days before finishing up in hospital

Ewan and Karen, taking a detour from where they had gone that morning, kindly offered to take us back from Menai Bridge to their warm cosy home, but Tom needed to plan an aspect of his wedding, having recently become engaged to Jo, and I needed to get back to see Dad.

By the time we got to McDonalds in Prestatyn, I was shivering violently, though some fluids and paracetamol improved matters.

Back at work, by the Monday afternoon, I took my temperature during surgery and it was 39°C, but I felt I could complete my surgery, not thinking I was particularly infectious. On the Wednesday Dad became acutely unwell with a chest infection, which I hoped I hadn't given him, and was admitted to hospital after the retirement home called the paramedics, where he gradually recovered over the following seven days.

By the Friday I felt increasingly unwell, more feverish, wheezy and weak, though fortunately that was on my day off. My GP kindly saw me, sent me for a chest X-ray, which was clear, took some bloods and prescribed antibiotics, an inhaler, and steroids because I was wheezy. My diabetes remained well controlled. I didn't go into work over the weekend, and felt a little better by the Monday. I went back to work, my teammates kindly covering urgent matters and any visits, and I didn't see anyone who was particularly vulnerable to infection. Mid March is still a particularly busy time in general medical practice, coming slowly out of winter, and I wanted to help out.

Dad was discharged on a Tuesday evening. Three months earlier, we had bought an adapted vehicle which I could drive, and wheel Dad inside in his wheelchair via a ramp at the back of the car. I had been too lazy to learn how to use the winch to pull the wheelchair in, as previously I had been able to push Dad in the wheelchair up the ramp. Dad, as ever, was non-complaining and extremely patient. It was eight o'clock in the evening, dark, cold, and raining, and try as I might I couldn't push Dad in, and I couldn't see how to use the winch. I thought I was going to cough my oesophagus up.

Fortunately a kind-hearted visitor helped me push Dad in, and off we went to the retirement village. Dad was dried off and well looked after by his excellent carers, who said I should go home to bed, which I did.

A few hours later, at around one in the morning, I woke up

feeling as if my heart was bouncing all over the place. I took my pulse and realised I was in quite rapid atrial fibrillation (AF). However, I had no chest pain or dizziness and didn't feel too bad otherwise, so I took my pills in the pocket and tried unsuccessfully to go back to sleep.

By five in the morning, I thought, stupidly, I may as well be at work, because it was my administration (catching up) day, where I didn't usually do face-to-face consultations.

I took another pill in the pocket, my usual other medications and went to work, but by seven o'clock in the morning, standing at my workstation, I was beginning to feel unwell.

Jean kindly saw me and performed an ECG which confirmed ongoing, moderately rapid AF, and then Rachel also saw me, later telling me that I looked an interesting shade of grey.

John helpfully insisted he take me to hospital, where I was admitted to the medical assessment unit. A couple of our recent Foundation Year 2 doctors made me feel very welcome.

Then I was transferred to the cardiac unit, where my pill in the pocket was tried in an intravenous form, with little effect. That evening, I heard that one of the consultant cardiologists, who works harder than I do, was going to discuss cardioverting me the next morning.

Sure enough, he amicably suggested cardioversion was the way forward, and after signing the consent form, I was shown into a very technical-looking side room. I was given an injection of midazolam, or at least I think it was that, my mind was still on how odd my chest felt. This is a highly effective sedative drug.

The next thing I knew, I was waking up back in the main ward, in normal sinus rhythm, having had a moderate amount of electricity sent through my heart via pads adhered to my chest. Apparently one does jump a little when the shock is given, but I felt no ill effects at all.

It was lovely to see Carole, Tom, Rachel and John who visited me, and that evening I was discharged. Needless to say, I felt rather foolish and behaved myself resting at home, taking even more pills daily. Fortunately, the other tests run in hospital did not show any underlying disease; perhaps just a basic lack of common sense!

I was now at about my ideal running weight, but I worried that I might not be able to run again. However, since my arrhythmia has never come on with exercise, three months later my cardiologist said I could. Phew!

I had already made one attempt, while wired up to a 24-hour ECG monitor. Actually, strictly speaking I'd taken another brief sprint, after I forgot to give Molly's food and water bowls to the man from Barking Mad who was taking her to a host home for a holiday before we went to Tenerife at the end of March. I legged it down the A49 shouting and carrying two metal dog bowls. Fortunately I caught up with him at the traffic lights, then felt rather like Andy Pipkin, the character from *Little Britain*, and went back to my sedate pace.

By early April I was feeling much better, and rather a fraud. I almost found myself watching *Emmerdale,* so I knew the time had come to go back to work (no offence to *Emmerdale* fans). My batteries felt recharged, appropriately enough after a cardioversion. My family, friends, and colleagues insisted I had a phased return, which was a good idea, so I didn't get up to speed until early May.

25. Tragedy.

Any problems I was experiencing were insignificant to what happened in Manchester on 22 May 2017. On the 21st, a friend and I had gone to the Manchester Arena to see Professor Brian Cox, which, for we nerdy types, was very interesting. The only hiccup apparently was that a group of Flat Earth Society members had been protesting outside. We left the show to the sound of the American band R.E.M. playing 'It's the end of the world as we know it'.

For many young people and their families the next day it really was the end of their world as they knew it, as an evil terrorist detonated a suicide bomb at the end of a pop concert. It shows how heinous these terrorists are; instead of targeting old geeks like me, the victims were innocent young people, many of whose lives had barely begun. Sickening beyond words.

26. Going Home.

Work was fairly full on during the summer, as at my instigation I tried to 'sort everybody out' before I retired. Again, not possible.

Colleagues and patients were very kind, touchingly saying they were sorry to see me go, but pleased for me and my family.

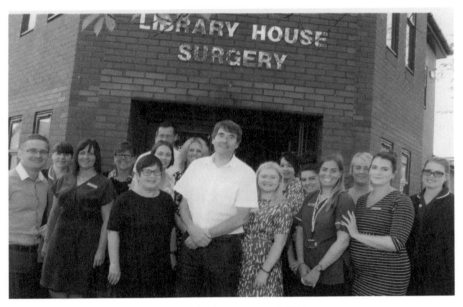

Outside the surgery, 2017

A 67-year-old lady accidentally referred to me as Dr Platt, partly because he and I were just about the only doctors she had ever had.

Movingly, there were a few tears. One doesn't become part of people's lives for over 30 years, sometimes during their most difficult phases, without making some sort of impact, hopefully usually for the better.

I used to get quite a few calls from Dad during surgery hours, when he was confused, which of course I answered, my patients being very understanding, and many people regularly enquired how he, Carole and the lads were.

I tried to get up to date with financial matters including my accounts. One sunny summer weekend morning, I almost found myself doing my tax returns instead of taking Molly for a walk first. It was just as well I was retiring. I was becoming like the father in the film *Shirley Valentine*, where the son says to him, 'You haven't half become a boring bastard'.

One of our friends said that in business there is a phrase 'gliding towards retirement'. Mine felt rather like hurtling kamikaze style, but sure enough on Thursday, 31 August 2017 I reached my last day of exactly 31 years as a GP Partner.

My last adult patient, a lady aged 87, attended with her daughter. I asked how I could help, and she said 'I'm slowing down'. I gave her a big smile and said something like 'brilliant'. She wasn't accepting that at 87 one slows down. She still wanted to be as active and lead as full a life as in years gone by.

My last afternoon, was, at my request, a child health surveillance clinic, where mums and dads bring their eight-week-old babies for a routine check-up. Seeing young families is quintessentially general medical practice, and my last patient was the daughter of a nice young man who was ever so grateful to me for seeing his daughter. I felt grateful too, for the privilege of my last consultation having been with them.

My last email to colleagues that day was titled 'School's Out'. I reckon I spent over 50,000 hours in that room, carried out over 200,000 face-to-face consultations in my career as a GP, and still hadn't got it right!

I thanked them for the privilege of working with them, and logged off from the computer. Getting into Virgil, I pressed the Number 2 button above the model cockpit, which I used to do on a Friday evening, to hear: 'This is Thunderbird 2. Mission complete, I'm on my way home.'

27. Lancashire Lad.

Carole and I are very settled in Chorley and don't plan to move for some time, and it is very unlikely we will move far.

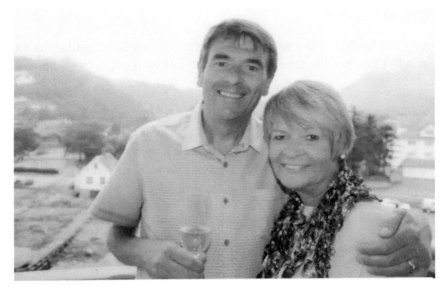

Carole and me

Although some people joke that families from Chorley and the surrounding villages don't venture far out of Lancashire, or indeed out of Chorley and the surrounding villages for that matter, many do. Indeed Myles Standish, possibly born in nearby Duxbury Hall, was on the *Mayflower* in 1620, to what is now North America.

Chorley is in fact an easy place to leave, being enclosed by the M6 to the west, M61 to the east and M65 to the north.

Manchester and Liverpool are barely 30 miles south, and Preston 10 miles north.

Chorley has people of many ethnic backgrounds. After World

War II, and more recently, Polish families settled here, and we also have families from Pakistan, India, China, Thailand, and Sri Lanka.

I have learned a lot from patients who themselves have come to live in England, or whose parents or grandparents did. I have enjoyed learning about their fascinating heritage, and occasionally receiving kind gifts from their lands of origin.

I have always tried to respect patients' psychological, spiritual, social, and cultural needs, and hope I have never let my opinions influence management.

Although in the last census over 90% of the population were White British, people from all ethnicities seem to get on well here, and work hard.

We have places of worship for the Church of England, Catholic and Methodist churches, a Mormon temple, a mosque, and a Jehovah's Witness hall. I have tried to become better informed about how religious and cultural factors can affect people's medical needs, for example, Ramadan and patients with diabetes.

In many areas of the country, language difficulties can make consultations more complex, but in Chorley most people seem to speak pretty good English, or have a family member or friend who can, at least the Lancashire version.

The bus station in Chorley has a huge slogan above it saying 'Lancashire, a place where everyone matters', and I am very proud now to call myself a Lancashire lad. Chorley is a great place to live, with great opportunities, and indeed a recent study showed that Chorley is the most economically mobile town in Lancashire.

28. Saying Goodbye.

In the weeks up to leaving, I was lucky enough to receive around 250 cards and several presents in the form of vouchers, gifts, cash or cheques, which was truly humbling. It's necessary, though, to be careful and open, particularly when receiving money, the majority of which I forwarded to the Motor Neurone Disease Association, with our patients' permission. The GMC is very clear that any gifts, particularly money, must not be seen as some form of financial inducement, for example, to treat someone differently. Since I was leaving, this could hardly be the case and I am truly grateful.

Again, I received lots of bottles of wine, and I intend to continue my 'lifelong learning' in this important field. Supplies are holding out, as even in retirement I am still trying not to drink during the week, with the emphasis on 'trying'.

The Chorley Guardian and *Lancashire Evening Post* were kind enough to run an article about my retiring. This may seem rather vain of me to have contacted them, but I wanted to thank all those patients I hadn't recently seen for their support over the years. I didn't realise I'd appear in the electronic version, and there were some kind comments on the Facebook page. I presume the less kind ones were vetted then deleted.

I have actually learned quite a lot from some of the comments and the cards I received, and though the following may seem massively conceited, I thought I'd put some of these remarks in this book. The reason for this is that I didn't realise some of the things I had done had made an impact, and that others following careers in healthcare, or indeed any field, or life in general, may be interested in what helps people.

'Care, compassion and dignified support', though I'm not so sure about the 'dignified'! This was written in a card showing a pea-

cock, which apparently is a symbol of integrity, guidance, protection and watchfulness, '*all the characteristics of a great GP!*'

'*You have been the backbone of my family's life. [My husband's] last words were about you*' – and I don't think those last words were 'if he had been a better doctor I wouldn't be this way'.

'*If ever a man found his vocation it was you*'.

'*You have helped me and guided me through so much, from being a scared, very young mum…*'.

'*Twelve years ago my dad was ill with cancer and my mum dementia. I was trying to look after both of them. You won't even remember this but you did a house call to check on Dad. Just as you were leaving you asked me how I was coping. This was so stunning. You were the only professional to say anything like this*'. Whether I was or not, I'm not sure, perhaps I just asked more loudly, as is my way. Now we are all acutely aware of carers' needs. '*Both Mum and Dad passed away years ago, but I have always remembered that small act of kindness. Sometimes words are better than medication!!*'

Other cards were touching for different reasons, such as a montage of little photos of a family of five I had looked after for almost a generation. Some families I had looked after for even longer. Mums and dads coming in with their kids, the parents themselves not having been born when I first started.

Some cards were from patients with whom the doctor/patient relationship had been strained at times, including those with substance misuse problems, for whom I had declined to prescribe what they were requesting.

Others recall events I didn't, including perhaps 'assuring me that all will be fine' to a lady during her pregnancy. This may have been premature, but fortunately all turned out well 25 years ago, after we listened into Baby's heartbeat at 16 weeks.

'Empathy and understanding' seem to be the main qualities to have, even though sometimes we can't fully understand what people are going through.

Although I didn't mention this in my first book, I have since reflected regarding what might have been my earliest effort at being empathic, and what perhaps subconsciously made me think I could go into healthcare.

A few schoolmates and I had gathered at the house of one of our friends. His father tragically had been killed, after stopping his car to remove a brick from the road. He'd been hit by another car. His mum was in another downstairs room. At 16 or 17 I had no idea what to say, but through the door, which stood ajar, I could see her looking sad. I went in and talked to her. I don't know what we said, but it seemed to help a little.

Since then I have said some crass and insensitive things when trying to help, sometimes so much so that silence would have been better on those occasions.

On balance it is probably better to say something, even just 'I'm sorry about your loss'.

In the last year I read an article in a medical journal saying how it is easy to be a popular doctor, but harder to be a good one. This I agree with. While as far as I'm aware I have never acceded to inappropriate requests, for example for medication or medical certificates, I have usually given patients the benefit of the doubt. More than one colleague has in the past suggested I need to say 'no' more, and Adam even bought me a book entitled *The Power of No*.

On one occasion, the context of which I forget, I said to Max that sometimes we need to say 'no', to which he replied, 'What a hypocrite'!

In the current climate of sexual harassment revelations, I sometimes wonder about the occasional hug or kiss I have received, usually from ladies in their eighties, but occasionally younger. Sometimes during consultations I have put my hand on a patient's hand or forearm to try to console them if they are distressed or upset, both male and female. I am not sure if current guidance would say this is wise, but for me, and my patients, it seemed instinctive.

29. Learning and Teaching.

If I could write a third book about what comes next, it might be called *A Way of Life and Death*, but since I doubt I'll be able to communicate after I have expired, I probably won't get chance. Perhaps *A Way of Life after Medicine* may be better. I do miss my colleagues and patients, but I do not miss getting up between four and five in the morning, and being knackered all the time. The real revelation is having time. Time to write this, time to be with Carole and the lads, and Dad, and time to go for a run. It's good not to feel rushed.

For the first three weeks I couldn't slow down. Actually, that's not strictly true. I slowed down for a day on the Sunday after I retired, after I'd been lucky enough to enjoy a good send-off. On a Friday we had a lunch where previous colleagues kindly came to join current ones, and Suzanne and her family organised a PowerPoint presentation, showing lots of embarrassing photos from over the years. I was also lucky enough to receive a number of presents, including, at my request, a voucher for a specialist walking shop where I could get boots adapted for my bunions.

I also gave back the seven keys and a fob that I would no longer need for the surgery, leaving me with only four keys and a fob for life outside work – and two of those were for Dad.

On the Saturday, we had a party, ably arranged by Patti, who is heroically typing this book, and her daughter Lauren. Hence the Sunday was rather quiet, as I had whiplash and was hoarse from playing and singing along to my air guitar.

On the Monday morning I went for an informal interview with the postgraduate tutors at the Royal Preston hospital, who were very understanding when I told them why I was hoarse and still holding my head asymmetrically.

A few weeks previously I had, with the help of Carole and our sons, drawn up my first CV for 31 years, and sent it, uninvited, to a number of places including the under- and postgraduate departments of medical education at the Preston deanery at the Royal Preston hospital, and the medical school at the University of Central Lancashire (UCLAN), in case I could be of any use to them and give something back.

They both kindly took me up, and I do ad hoc teaching sessions, some voluntary and some paid. Needless to say on my part they are not high-tech, and I still couldn't put together a PowerPoint presentation if my life depended on it.

Some are informal talks about aspects of general practice. On one occasion I asked a group of about 30 Foundation Year 2 doctors if any of them were thinking of a career in general practice. Four sheepishly raised their hands. I've tried to be enthusiastic and encourage them at least to consider the options general medical practice can offer, hopefully conveying that the advantages significantly outweigh any disadvantages.

Other sessions are small-group work, mainly helping with communication skills, and I am pleased to say tomorrow's doctors seem to have a good grasp of what it takes to talk with someone as a person, rather than as a collection of symptoms. This seems to be in part because of much better emphasis on the consultation than in my early days as a medical student or doctor. The Calgary–Cambridge model is used, consisting of: initiating the session; gathering information; physical examination where needed; explanation and planning; and then closing a session; all the while providing structure and building the doctor/patient relationship during a consultation. In my subsequent years the importance of recognising the patient's ideas, concerns and expectations was the focus, and I have heard of young doctors in general practice writing 'ICE' on the inside of the surgery door to remind them, particularly when consultations were videoed, making sure this prompt was out of the filming field. In recent years I've been interested to learn various mnemonics such as SPIKES, for example when breaking bad news. S – Setting up the consultation; P – assessing patient's Perception (what the person understands is happening already); I – obtaining a patient's Invitation to share information. (For example, 'Would you like me to give you all the information now, or would you like me to give you an outline of the test results and perhaps spend more time later discussing a treatment plan?'). This varies from patient to patient and situation to situation. K – giving Knowledge and information to the patient; E – address the patient's emotions with Empathy; and S – a Strategy and summary. Usually a clear plan will reduce anxiety.

At medical school I don't recall one session being offered on medical ethics. Possibly we had just one on breaking bad news. I don't think that tomorrow's doctors will have the temerity to say to a patient or relatives 'there's nothing we can do', as patients in my generation of doctors have been told, though never by me. There is always something we can do to help even if there is no cure. We can comfort, support, and alleviate symptoms. One of my patients was told by a neurologist that she had motor neurone disease. She stoically asked what the prognosis was, and he said he hadn't time to discuss that now!

As well as teaching, I was going to do locum sessions elsewhere, and was lucky enough to be offered work, but after three months of careful consideration the thought of working with less familiar colleagues, patients with whom it would be less easy to establish continuity (and make safety-netting phone calls to at silly hours in the morning), and figure out unfamiliar IT and operation systems, has made me decide against it.

I will remain registered with the GMC, BMA, Royal College of General Practitioners (RCGP), and a medical indemnity organisation, but I am giving up my licence to practise medicine with patients.

This is a big step for me and one not taken lightly. For over 40 years my aim has been to learn and to try to help people, in the privileged position of doctor.

I still hope to help people, particularly to learn from my experiences; both good ones and those where things have gone less well, just as I have learned from colleagues and patients over the years. That is partly why I am writing this book.

When one of my patients learned of my retirement he told me a story about one of his colleagues in the Post Office, who had been diagnosed with terminal cancer in his mid sixties just after his retirement. The dying man said to his friend, my patient, who was in his mid fifties at the time, 'If you don't retire at sixty, I'll come back and haunt you.'

If my dad had retired at 65, he and my mum would have had two years together before she developed MND.

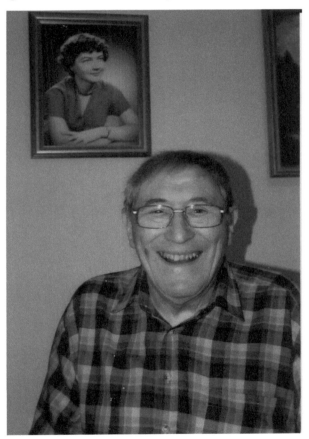

My Dad, 2017, in his apartment. The picture behind is of my Mum on her 21st birthday, around the time they met

I am acutely aware that I am lucky to be able to retire from my lifelong vocation at 58½ years old. Many of you reading this will need to work into your mid or even late sixties to benefit financially from a full pension. Again, I am aware that NHS pensions for my generation are significantly more generous than today's, though I have paid a quarter of my income into it for many years.

I would respectfully suggest that readers of this book and others try not to work full-time into their sixties, or at least not work as many hours as I did in the decade before.

In recent months I have reflected on my work patterns. I can better see that I may have overdone it. The wife of one of my close friends, herself a senior nurse, said at times she had felt like a one-parent family. Carole wishes I had been around more when the lads were growing up, and so do I. Rarely, if ever, has anyone been heard to say at the end of their life, 'I wish I'd worked more.'

30. Gap Life.

Three weeks after leaving Library House, Carole and I went on a sort of 'gap life' inter-railing trip, through Holland, Belgium, and north east France. This was a really good idea because I couldn't feel I should always be doing something, like I did at home, from sending emails to sorting the sock drawer. I still don't have a smartphone, so unless someone contacted us on the emergency phone numbers we had provided, we could just chill.

We sat outside inns and restaurants, ate and drank, watched people and the world go by, and walked hand in hand around Amsterdam and Bruges and Rouen and everywhere. Phew!

My weeks now begin with an hour's yoga class, courtesy of a patient who became a friend.

I am a little more bendy than I was when I started, though I still struggle with various positions, including the 'downward facing dog', thanks to my weedy arms. It's also just as well my shoulder is fixed, as in earlier times I would have dislocated it within minutes of starting a session. I have even managed not to fart loudly in the more buttock-straining positions.

Carole quite rightly suggests plumbing, carpentry, or bricklaying lessons may be more productive, but I do enjoy yoga.

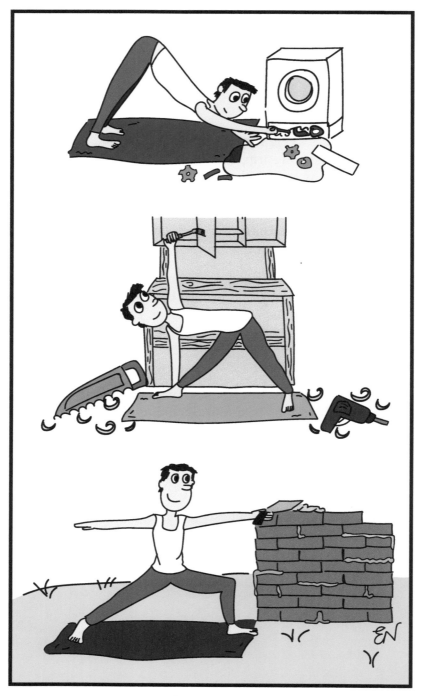

Extreme Yoga

I run at least once a week including occasional Saturday morning park runs (parkrun.org.uk), where it's great to see mass participation sport. My targets for the coming year are 5k in 25 minutes, 10k in 55 minutes, and half-marathons in 2 hours 10 minutes. These are hardly 'good for age' times, and are certainly not a pretty sight. Even though my weight is steady at 11½ stones (BMI 22), I still finish very sweaty and red-faced, and due to either my medical conditions or treatment or both, I seem to foam at the mouth. I'm trying to run a half-marathon every month in 2018.

I will retire from marathon-running after London 2019, which will also be my last major fundraising event. People have been very generous over the years, including many of you reading this book.

Tom, Adam and I plan to raise £10,000 for the Motor Neurone Disease Association by running the 26 miles 385 yards that is the London Marathon in April 2019. I will be 60 years old on 7 March, six weeks before. As the saying goes, 'If your dreams don't scare you, they aren't big enough'.

I feel a lot healthier than I did this time a year ago. My heart is behaving itself and my diabetes is better controlled. I feel more relaxed, and I'm grinding my teeth less. Some years ago I tried wearing a splint at night to reduce the speed at which my teeth disintegrated, and to reduce headaches and neck pain, but I couldn't get used to it. From Carole's description of some of my nocturnal upper respiratory symptoms, I sound like a warthog being strangled. At times I have accused Carole of snoring when she is simply breathing and is in fact awake, but I have been such a light sleeper since my junior hospital doctor days I'm easily distracted from sleep.

One of my friends who we initially got to know as a patient kindly gave me *The Little Book of Mindfulness* three years ago, and although some people are sceptical about mindfulness (for example the recent re-working of the Ladybird books, for adults, which are admittedly very funny), I have found being mindful very helpful. Focussing on what one is experiencing *now* is usually beneficial for most people.

On a couple of occasions we have been to our friends Mike and Diane's home where the musician Francis Dunnery was performing a house concert. He has also researched in psychology, and I took note of his thoughts about not living in the future, where one can become anxious, nor living in the past, where one can become depressed, but living in the now. Obviously if one is in the nightmare scenarios where something terrible is happening in the world, then now is not a good place to be, but for most of us here it's okay, or indeed a lot better than okay.

I do still have diurnal variation sometimes, when I wake up feeling a little anxious and asking myself why I committed myself to something the day or two before. Then within hours I am excited, and up for anything.

My achievements and aspirations are small compared to some but we can all have them, even if we don't make it to who we thought we might be at the beginning of our lives; in my case, as I noted at the start of my first book, an astronaut or a rock star.

The nearest I got to being an astronaut was gazing in wonder at the Saturn 5 rocket at the Kennedy Space Centre in Florida some years ago. On our study wall I have a signed photograph of Buzz Aldrin standing on the moon, with Neil Armstrong and the lunar module reflected in his visor. Carole is concerned that if we had a fire at home I would rescue Buzz before anyone or anything else. As for being a rock star, I almost reached Grade 1 piano aged 12, and learnt to play the chord E on the guitar. Other than that it has been my air guitar, or occasional appalling singing in karaoke.

I would like to go on for a few years and be around for Carole, Tom, Adam and Max, Dad and others if possible. I realise I have had more years of good health than many people are lucky enough to get, so if in my case that doesn't happen, so be it.

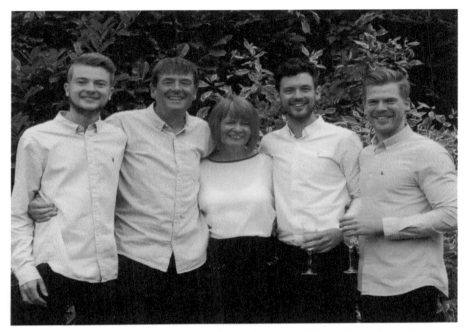

The five of us 2016 (My head is rather red 'cos we'd been in the lake district that day and I'd been photographing the lads in a 'Total Warrior' 10k obstacle course. They'd been covered in mud, but I got burnt!)

We recently attended the 35-year graduation reunion from Manchester medical school and a significant number of our year attended. Some couldn't be contacted, some couldn't make it, and some have already died. My great friends and housemates from nearly 40 years ago, Ewan, Danny, and Graham, and I have been 'volunteered' to organise the 40-year reunion. We have all been wonderfully supported by our wives; Karen, Jane, Avril, and Carole. In fact at the 20-year reunion the senior manager of the medical school, Harry, started his speech by saying, 'Would the following please stand up: Mrs Thomas, Mrs McAllister, Mrs Hazelhurst, and Mrs Barker.' Our ladies stood up apprehensively, and Harry turned to them and said, 'You poor things, how do you manage?'!

I think I've still got all my faculties, though I do now make a weekly list to remind me of things I am supposed to be doing. I understand some people do this on their smartphones. I then usually lose my list somewhere, and make a second list for that week, the first task being 'find first list'!

One of my patient's cards depicted a retirement class, with a teacher showing a pie chart on the blackboard, and saying, 'We can see from the example on the board how each day can be divided into different activities'. Almost half the pie chart was a section reading, 'Searching for things you only put down a minute ago'. I know the feeling already, and if I become confused or demented, please ignore anything I say. I already talk to myself, or give running commentaries of what I am doing, particularly cooking, at which I'm still hopeless. I also whistle or sing badly, or apparently repeat inane phrases such as 'there we go'.

Now that I have more time and am less tired, I try to be more attentive to what Carole and other people are saying. Eighteen months ago I went for a hearing test, to see if we could clarify whether I couldn't hear well, or wasn't listening. Unfortunately it turned out I wasn't listening! In recent years when out with Molly I have walked past people I knew without acknowledging them, as my brain was so full of thoughts whizzing around. Now I am more aware; mindful, in fact.

31. The Future.

Where we'll go next, I'm not quite sure. We've asked the lads about their experiences, and the most exhilarating seems to be a free-fall tandem parachute jump, and the most frightening, a bungie jump. Carole is thinking about the parachute jump attached to some hunky Antipodean, and I'm thinking about a bungie jump in New Zealand, though with my back and heart history, I'm not sure if they'd take me.

One of my patients who has become a friend is a pest controller, and he says he's going to take me on an extreme wasp or bee experience this year. Even our lads haven't done that!

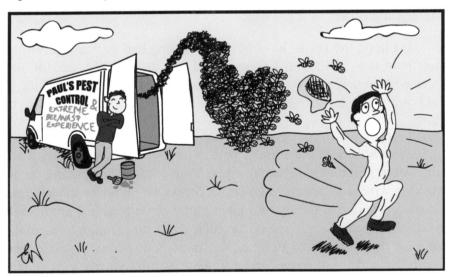

Gap Life Adventures

My most recent running friend is a colleague I've known for many years, who is a consultant psychiatrist, which is probably quite appropriate. As I have written, read, and re-written and re-read this book, I have become aware that the narrative is rather all over the place, mixing work with life supposedly outside work and vice versa.

I suppose this is because each impacts on the other and the boundaries between life and medicine blur, hence the title of my books. In fact it probably seems that I have 'flight of ideas', one definition of which is 'a rapid shifting of ideas with only superficial associative connections between them that is expressed as a disconnected rambling from subject to subject and occurs especially in the manic phase of bipolar disorder'.

It is just possible, depending on how uninhibited I am when this book is published, that I might do a little talk at a small local venue if they'll allow me. If so, I'd love to see you there.

I am aware when writing this that I am still referring to myself as a doctor, which as I'm still registered with the GMC is in order, but I am no longer in clinical practice with patients. If I was, I wouldn't have time to write this! I respect those people still working in medicine, healthcare, and indeed any walk of life contributing to society and helping others in some way.

I hope the books have been interesting and perhaps helpful in their own way. Although I appear loud and confident, I am not, and there will be times when I ask myself why did I not put something in the book that I should have, and at other times think, 'Why did I write that?'

Tom said, at least once, with Adam and Max agreeing, that I am 'living the dream'. They're right. I have had a fascinating career working with and for amazing people, for which I have been well paid. I have a wonderful family and have pretty good health. I am acutely aware that many people are not so lucky, and that although hopefully some of my 'luck' is of my making, most of it is due to others: my family; friends; colleagues and patients, in other words, you. Thank you, and as we yogis say, *namaste*.

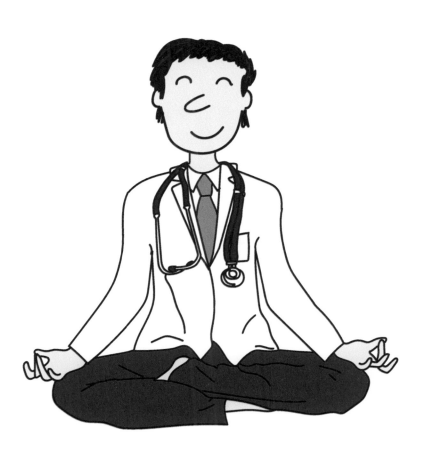

BV - #0055 - 190219 - C25 - 229/152/9 - CC - 9781909607187